ADAPTIVE
TRAINING

ADAPTIVE TRAINING

Building a Body
That's Fit
for Function

ADAM SINICKI

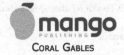

mango
PUBLISHING

CORAL GABLES

For permission requests, please contact the publisher at:
Mango Publishing Group
2850 S Douglas Road, 4th Floor
Coral Gables, FL 33134 USA
info@mango.bz

For special orders, quantity sales, course adoptions and corporate sales, please email the publisher at sales@mango.bz. For trade and wholesale sales, please contact Ingram Publisher Services at customer.service@ingramcontent.com or +1.800.509.4887.

Adaptive Training: Building a Body That's Fit for Function

Library of Congress Cataloging-in-Publication number: 2022944397
ISBN: (print) 978-1-68481-112-0, (ebook) 978-1-68481-113-7
BISAC category code: HEA015000, Health &Fitness/Men's Health

Printed in the United States of America

This book is dedicated to my amazing family: my two wonderful children, Emmy and Alex, and my incredible wife, Hannah. I love you guys!

Also, a massive shout-out to my friend and frequent collaborator, Grant Stevens, who has the same passion for this kind of stuff as I do and has been a huge support in growing the channel.

And to every gym buddy whose friendships were forged in iron, alphabetically: Chris "Goof" Hanlon, Janik Rajapakse, Nathan Wallace, and Simon Dowe.

Oh, and to my subscribers. I'm incredibly lucky to have the most supportive and positive comments section on all of YouTube. I'm not sure what I did to deserve it—I'm a guy who pretends to be Batman for a living—but I'm eternally grateful.

And to the team at Mango Publishing for giving me a second go-round and making this book possible!

And to you, dear reader. Cheers to that.

Table of Contents

INTRODUCTION

What are the limits of human performance?

What can we achieve through training?

And how can we overcome setbacks and shortcomings to feel our best?

These are some of the questions I've obsessed over for far too long now.

Through my education in psychology and fitness, my career as a health and fitness writer, and now as "The Bioneer," I've spent decades researching the best ways to enhance human performance. I've been hugely fortunate to have met and trained with some truly incredible athletes, spoken to some of the best coaches and fitness influencers, and learned about some incredible outliers that push the boundaries of what's physically possible. I've consumed absurd amounts of literature and written several books.

And I've spent thousands of hours in the gym, training myself and others, testing the ideas and techniques I've discovered.

Turns out, I may have been barking up the wrong tree. Perhaps what we do in the gym isn't quite as important as I had presumed.

Huh.

It is natural to think that we can take control of our physical health through training. We can choose to build muscle, gain mobility, or lose weight by spending more time at the gym with the appropriate program.

Though such attempts are admirable and certainly can be effective, they are often not enough. We are not our training. Rather, we are the products of our environments, routines, and habits.

Or at least, this is what I have come to conclude.

Even if you ran ten kilometres three times a week, that would only be around 1,800 calories burned. That's not even a day's worth of calories for most people.

The number of curls you perform in your life will never come *close* to the number of keystrokes you make.

This leads to the logical conclusion: everything else you do outside of training is more important.

What you do *regularly* is much more important than what you do sporadically.

The same goes for our mobility, strength, and mental agility. If all you do is sit on the sofa, then sit at work, no amount of training at the gym can undo that damage.

Likewise, we must think of our training in the context of our lifestyles outside of the gym. It's impossible to tease this apart; someone who has a laid-back lifestyle will find their recovery time is different from someone who works a physical job and then looks after three kids when they get home.

To ignore the role of your environment and lifestyle in training is to invite disappointment and failure.

It's not a matter of our environment being the bigger stimulus, though. It's also the fact that we are *built* to adapt to our environments. This is *why* our bodies are capable of change in the first place: to help us to respond to the changing demands of the world around us—to improve our chances of survival.

Natural selection has little interest in sixteen-inch biceps or washboard abs. It doesn't care about how great you can get at football.

It cares about how efficiently you can complete the tasks you need to complete every day.

By understanding this, we can potentially tap into a *far* greater plastic potential. If we understand how the body can respond to environmental demands, we can understand how to trigger the changes we want.

When we see that the body is built to respond to the environment's frequency, variability, and challenges, we discover new ways to elicit massive change. Not only that, but we can trigger this change *without* spending huge amounts of time performing dull and repetitious movements.

Ultimately, the best way to train our bodies is to stop "training" them and *live* the way we want to perform.

There is no better gym than your environment. No better coach than the challenges you face daily.

That's my thesis, anyway. Now it's my job to convince you and lay out a practical strategy to make that happen...

Chapter 1

YOUR AMAZING, ADAPTABLE BODY

You're pretty amazing, really. You know that, right?

I don't even know you, but I can safely make this assumption because you're *human*. And as a human, you have limitless, adaptable potential.

Nice one, mate.

This is something we rarely stop to consider. But the journey we took to get here and the destination we arrived at…it's all truly incredible.

And this incredible adaptability and resilience give us such infinite potential to change and improve our bodies and minds.

Your Journey Through Space

Let's start with the basics.

As a human, you are a carbon-based lifeform. Carbon is formed in the hearts of dying stars. The core of a red giant is compressed until the forces are great enough to start fusing helium nuclei together.

Once the carbon in your body was born, it travelled countless light years through space to end up on Earth and become *you*.

But, of course, it was many other things before it was you. The same carbon atoms that make up your body were once a part of other animals, plants, and who knows what else. Maybe dinosaurs. Maybe aliens!

Those carbon atoms make up the approximately 37.2 trillion cells inside your body right now.

But what's even more spectacular is that every one of those cells will be replaced within the next ten years. Like the ship of Theseus, everything that physically comprises "you" will be replaced. And yet "you" will remain.

So, you are more than the atoms that create your body. You are literally more than the sum of your parts.

We must assume, then, that the information truly matters. That vital data is carried with you as DNA—an identical genetic code found in the nuclei of all those trillions of cells.

Your Incredible DNA

Just one gram of DNA could store up to 215 petabytes of information. That's 215 million gigabytes or three billion "units" of information.[1]

To put it another way, you could install *Doom Eternal* on your DNA 2,687,500 times.

---

1   *Mapping and Sequencing the Human Genome*, National Academies Press.

The gulf between biology and human technology may be truly insurmountable.[2]

Perhaps surprisingly, 99.9 percent of this data—this DNA—is identical across all humans. In fact, humans share 50 percent of their DNA with bananas!

You are half a banana.

This is more understandable when we consider how related we are. You and I are at least fiftieth cousins. I know this because that is generally the most distantly related you can be from anyone on Earth.

In your region, it's highly likely you're far more related to much of the population.

Where did you meet your current partner again?

We're also highly related to every animal on Earth. In fact, we are all descendants of LUCA: the Last Universal Common Ancestor that emerged on Earth four billion years ago.[3]

Each of those genes is a stretch of DNA that encodes a specific function or trait (admittedly, a simplification). The gene instructs the creation of a protein at a specific location. On a macroscopic level, that is what builds a human.

There are roughly 30,000 of these in the human genome, stored as twenty-three pairs of chromosomes (the twenty-third being the sex

---

2   This is why I think computers in the distant future will be biological.

3   Or are we? If we were ever to find life that was not a part of this family tree, it would be evidence of what's referred to as the "shadow biosphere." In other words: life on Earth is as distant from humans as an extra-terrestrial would be! Some believe such life forms indeed exist, inhabiting Earth's most inhospitable places. Maybe even magma.

chromosomes). Chromosomes carry near-identical sequences but differ in a few places where unique traits (alleles) are inherited from different parents. Here we will see the "dominant" gene expressed, or the two will interact in some way.

Since 99.9 percent of DNA is identical across humans, most interest is placed on the genes that differ more often. These commonly changeable positions are called "single nucleotide polymorphisms." To classify as such, they must vary in more than 1 percent of the population.[4] We call these SNPs or "snips."

Countless studies show how specific SNPs correlate with particular traits. Some of these might determine things like eye colour. Others might give you a competitive advantage in sports. For example, the ACTN3 gene (SNP rs1815739) encodes the protein alpha-actinin-3, which results in greater fast twitch muscle fiber and, therefore, greater power-based athleticism.[5]

More on this later.

Some of these differences may surprise you. For example: did you know that we don't all have the same muscles? Certain muscles only exist in a percentage of the population. And this is normal!

For example, 20 percent of the population lacks the triangular abdominal muscle called the "pyramidalis." That's just one example.

Should this affect the way we train?

---

4   Rarer variants are called mutations.

5   Nan Yang et al., "ACTN3 genotype is associated with human elite athletic performance," Am J Hum Genet 73, no. 3 (2003): 627–31.

We're All X-Men

What's perhaps even more exciting is that all of us are mutants.

Genetic mutations are changes to the DNA sequence that are considered abnormal or extremely rare. While it's expected that our eyes vary in colour, you'd be surprised if your *ears* were a different colour. That would be a mutation.

Beneficial mutations are rare by definition. After all, if they were beneficial, they would survive and make their way into the population. That said, they *do* occur. And they kind of make superheroes?

One famous example is the mutation affection the myostatin (MSTN) gene. Myostatin is a compound that *limits* muscle growth. In rare cases where this is down-regulated, individuals can experience "double muscling." That's pretty much what it sounds like: superior muscle strength and size, with increased running speed to go with it (at least in the case of whippet dogs).

Most mutations are harmful, however. Indeed, the MSTN mutation might also increase the likelihood of tendon injuries.

The surprising thing is that we all have genetic mutations that largely go unnoticed. We are all mutants.

And, as a side note, it is not only *our* DNA that we carry. Hitching a ride are countless bacteria that live inside our bodies, providing crucial roles like breaking down food and fighting off harmful invaders. We have a symbiotic relationship with these creatures, to the point that they are almost a part of us. They can even affect our mood.

We are not a single organism but a *superorganism*.

Not one, but many.

Indeed, some bacteria became a part of us billions of years ago. The mitochondria that live in our cells and help us to harness energy from our food began life as a separate form of alphaproteobacterial.

Thus, mitochondria have an entirely different set of DNA.

Gene Expression

While every cell in the body might carry identical DNA, the way DNA behaves is entirely different. This is due to "gene expression." Different genes within our code are active or inactive depending on their location in the body. This is how bone cells can act like bone cells and muscle cells like muscle cells.

The best way to imagine this is as a long list of random letters that always remains the same but where crossing out certain letters can form a wide range of words.

This is also how our bodies can change to a nearly infinite degree throughout our lives. Everything from diet to training to our *thoughts* can alter our gene expression—sometimes indefinitely. This can drastically impact our suitability for the environment around us.

We are not stuck playing the hand we are dealt.

And this allows even more variation than the initial 0.1 percent that separates us from one another at birth. This is where we can truly separate ourselves from the pack.

Your Amazing Brain

Perhaps the most complex and amazing part of the human body is the brain. The brain is comprised of over a hundred billion brain cells, which we call neurons. There are over 125 trillion synapses (connections) between these cells.

To put that in perspective, it's 1,500 times the number of stars in our galaxy.

This earns the brain its title as "the most complex known object in the universe."

So, look after yours!

The job of the brain and nervous system is to help us navigate our environment: to adapt and alter our behaviour and thus optimize our chances of survival.

To this end, it is capable of incredible change. The brain, we now know, is "plastic." Neuroplasticity is the ability of the brain to grow new connections and neurons and cull those it no longer needs.

So incredibly versatile is the human brain that it can retain most of its functions even after a hemispherectomy (where half the brain is removed).

Another incredible example of this plasticity is seen in individuals who develop "echolocation." Echolocation is the ability to "see" using sound, like a bat (or Daredevil). This "sonar" is achieved using clicks and whistles and is mostly experienced by those with impaired vision.

If it's possible to teach yourself to use sonar, imagine what else might be possible.

This plasticity doesn't only occur in response to severe trauma, however. It also occurs in response to our routines and daily activities. Your job may affect how you *think* and experience the world around you!

Did you know, for example, that wrestlers use different parts of their brain when mentally rotating 3D objects?[6] They rely less on their visual cortices and more on their kinaesthetic awareness—no doubt because they have become more in-tune with moving their body in 3D space.

Writers, likewise, may think differently from artists. How has your lifestyle impacted the way you think?

Meanwhile, the human brain is so incredibly powerful, capable of such unbelievable imagination, that single brains have created equations that accurately predict the behaviour of black holes and even the universe's shape through time.

And we have *zero* idea how our body generates consciousness. We have no idea how it can do this.

We Can Not Separate the Brain and Body

Far from being a brain in a vat, our experience is inexorably tied to our physicality. We may not even be able to *think* were it not for our bodies!

---

6   David Moreau, "The role of motor processes in three-dimensional mental rotation: Shaping cognitive processing via sensorimotor experience," *Learning and Individual Differences* 22 (2011): 354–359.

The theory of "embodied cognition" suggests that we use our bodies to understand the physical world. This is, perhaps, best exemplified by language. How do we *understand* language? What does the brain "translate" language into when it interprets it? What is the "base code" of the brain?

We may understand what people say to us by essentially "experiencing" it. We know that when listening to someone talk, brain areas light up that correspond to what's being said to us. If someone tells us how they opened the door, our premotor cortex fires as though *we* were opening a door.

At a more abstract level, even our understanding of maths is tied to our experience of quantities and counting.

It appears that the primary function of the nervous system is to navigate the environment and that our more abstract abilities are built on top of that.

So it is that the human body is capable of incredible, graceful, and powerful movement. In fact, it has been argued, by the likes of neuroscientist Daniel Wolpert, that movement is the brain's primary function.

The Miraculous Maths of Movement

We move to pick up a glass or bend over and tie our laces without thinking. But while this movement might seem simple on the surface, it is only possible thanks to a huge number of different inputs and calculations.

Your body must consider its current position in space: your current stance and your distance from the target object. It must then coordinate the movement of countless muscles to create the right amount of leverage and move at the right speed with perfect precision.

Move too fast and you might launch that cup across the room. Move too slowly and you'll be wasting precious time.

To do all this, the body listens to detailed feedback from a host of sensors. Not only do we use our balance (equilibrioception) and sight to plan our movement, but we also consider the lengths of each muscle. This is accomplished thanks to muscle spindles, which can sense the length of muscles alongside other proprioceptors like the Golgi tendon organs and Pacinian corpuscles. These sense changes in tension within the tendons, and pressure changes within the skin, respectively.

So much for seven senses!

The Fascia

Helping to coordinate all this movement is the fascia. The fascia has only recently become the focus of serious study but is increasingly thought to be an integral piece of the puzzle.

The fascia is a sheet of connective tissue that wraps around the entire body. More than a "catsuit," though, it also encapsulates and surrounds individual muscles and organs. It even penetrates the muscles creating separate segments like an orange. This aspect of the connective tissue is referred to as "epimysium," with the created segments known as "fascicles."

The amazing thing about fascia is that it is far more "alive" than you might reasonably presume. The fascia contains motor units, meaning it can generate force and proprioceptors.

What's more, is that these capabilities allow for even greater coordination and power. Fascial force generation explains muscle contraction in one area can trigger contraction elsewhere in the body. For this to happen, the fascial tissue must maintain constant tension throughout the entire system. This is known as "tensegrity."

Tensegrity

Simplified models of the human body, such as you might encounter when reading a biology textbook, depict the body as a series of hinges, pulleys, and levers. Each muscle has "one job," which is to enact action across a single joint.

An understanding of fascia and tensegrity, however, demonstrates this to be entirely insufficient.

As author James Earls explains in his book *Born to Walk*,[7] the primary job of the hip adductors is not to adduct the hips (bring them closer to the centre line). Rather, it is to *prevent* abduction. The adductors and the abductors are in constant balance, producing the body's resting state.

This same process occurs throughout the entire system and is what keeps us from flailing around wildly during movement. Were we a "stack of bones" piled on top of each other, rather than a tensegrity structure,

---

7   James Earls, *Born to Walk: Myofascial Efficiency and the Body in Movement* (West Sussex, England: Lotus Publishing, 2020).

we would collapse when leaning too far to one side. Our organs would
constantly drop into the wrong places.

Pretty gross.

We are less tower of blocks and more spiderweb.

And thanks to this, an increase in tension in the glute can travel across
the thoracolumbar fascia[8] and be felt in the lats. As the glute on one
side contracts, this tension is felt in the lats, triggering the movement
of the arms.

This movement can happen reflexively, with no need to make the long
and costly trip to the brain.

And this perfectly explains why damage to one muscle can result in pain
and compensatory movement patterns on the other side of the body.

The fascia, too, is plastic. Like the brain, the fascia can change its shape
and structure in response to its use. This occurs via fibroblast cells that lay
down collagen and collagenase in response to stress and pressure signals.

Your structure can alter itself to allow for optimal movement through
the environment.

Again, this allows us to adapt to changing environmental demands. This
is a common theme throughout the body. Even our *bones* can change
according to such demands. Whereas we often think of the bones as rigid
and unchanging, they act far more like "banks" for calcium and other
minerals that the body can draw on as needed.

---

8   Fascia that travels along the middle and bottom of the back.

Your Limitless Potential

I'm hoping that you take two things away from this chapter.

The first: you are a truly incredible specimen. The fact you exist is nothing short of a cosmic miracle. The intricacy of even your simplest function goes far beyond anything human technology could hope to fully understand, let alone replicate.

The second is you are also incredibly *adaptable*. We have evolved over countless generations to exist in synergy with our environment. But even within our lifetimes, we are capable of immense change at a physical level. Our brains can change shape and create new pathways. Our bones can be absorbed and rebuilt as necessary. Our muscles and fascia can restructure themselves.

Our DNA constantly rewrites itself like an author who can't let it be. Every cell in our body will be replaced multiple times during our lives.

This incredible changeability should be empowering. You can truly be what you want to be.

Your potential is unlimited.[9]

And the key to that potential is the environment you exist in.

---

9   Well done, you!

Chapter 2

CHANGE THE ENVIRONMENT, CHANGE THE ORGANISM

Sorry if that's a lot of pressure! If you find yourself sitting in your pants at eleven in the morning, surrounded by your mess (as I tend to be), you might not feel "limitless."

With all that incredible changeability and potential at our fingertips, how do we leverage it?

How do we steer the change and dictate our evolution?

Again, the answer is simple: we change the environment.

The environment is what has been guiding our development up to this point. Our body's *job* is to thrive under the conditions it is presented with, and it will continue to do this.

By changing our immediate environment, we can bring about a passive transformation within ourselves.

The problem? While the environment has an incredible ability to shape humans, humans also have an unprecedented ability to *shape the environment*. And unfortunately, we have succumbed to our base instincts when doing so.

Our impulse to make everything as comfortable, safe, and easy as possible has ironically damaged our bodies.

Look around the room you are in right now. The floor is likely flat. Anything you might conceivably need is likely not only within reach but also *at arm's length*. You don't even need to reach up or stoop down.

There are multiple soft places to sit.[10] You have little reason to walk more than a few steps until you run out of food and need to go to the shop.

Even then, you probably have enough supply to last you *weeks*.

Our man-made environment is not only making us soft but also de-training us. In some cases, and sorry to be so dramatic, it is *killing* us.

This is the main thesis of this book. I intend to demonstrate why the environment you create for yourself is *critical* in impacting your health and performance and present a methodology to make that happen.

I'm not talking about making yourself healthier. I'm talking about leveraging your surroundings to passively improve human performance exponentially.

And don't worry; it won't necessarily involve installing monkey bars into your ceiling.

Except yes, it will!

But also, not that. There are levels.

You'll get it.

---

10 How many chairs can you see right now?

How the Natural Environment Creates Powerful Humans

If you were to move out of your home right now and live instead in a forest, you would toughen up.

Now, you might die of pneumonia *first*. But were you to survive the initial…ah, *rough patch*, you would emerge tougher.

Like Green Arrow, for the comics fans out there. Or Tarzan, for the rest of you.

A tougher and more *varied* environment naturally shapes us more optimally.

Not for bodybuilding competitions or powerlifting, of course, but for healthy and normal movement. For joint longevity. And for efficient movement.

Now, I'm not here to tell you that all indigenous populations are incredibly fit and healthy. But it is clear to see how they have been able to adapt to their environments in incredible ways.

A popular example is that of the Rarámuri, or Tarahumara, tribe. This group of indigenous people living in Chihuahua, Mexico, are well-known for their amazing running abilities. In fact, the name *Rarámuri* means "runners on foot."

The Tarahumara are known to run huge distances, sometimes up to two hundred miles in a single session, spread over two days.[11]

---

11   Christopher McDougall, *Born to Run: A Hidden Tribe, Superathletes, and the Greatest Race the World Has Never Seen* (London, UK: Profile Books, 2009).

Many tribes of humans are capable of incredible free diving. For example, the Moken people get a huge amount of food from the bottom of the Andaman Sea. As such, they've adapted an ability to see clearly underwater by physically bending the lenses in their eyes to counter the refraction of water. They do this while narrowing their pupils to "the limits of human performance."

This skill can be taught to anyone—the Moken have no unique physical traits in this sense—but it only works for children.

The Bajau "Sea Nomads," meanwhile, are capable of diving to depths of seventy meters and holding their breath for thirteen minutes or more. In this case, evolution has caused physical changes: the Bajau have spleens that are 50 percent larger than other humans!

On land, indigenous members of Australia's "NORFORCE" unit have been reported to have "super sight." According to Professor Taylor from the University of Melbourne's Indigenous Eye Health Unit, some people have 6:14 vision. That means they can see what the average person sees from 1.4 meters away as clearly at six meters away!

These were the most exceptional individuals in the study, but nearly all the Aboriginal subjects had far better vision than the average person. The same Aboriginals could identify constellations that would otherwise require binoculars to view.

The "Twa" people are hunter-gatherers found in the rainforests of Uganda who climb trees to forage for food. Their tree-climbing abilities are incredibly impressive, especially given their short average height.

We can even observe the "head-carrying" capabilities of many cultures as extremely impressive. Some individuals can carry as much as 20 percent of their body weight on top of their heads without it negatively impacting their walking efficiency. This is possible as they can translate the downward force into elastic energy.

That, in turn, may be due to their exceptional posture and spinal health.

You'll often read the "indigenous cultures don't get back pain." This is a bit of a sweeping claim that isn't backed by enough evidence, but there is a grain of truth. It has even been suggested that sitting has incorrectly *altered* the shapes of our spines; we should feature "j" shaped spines rather than the "s" shape we're so familiar with.[12]

This is a somewhat controversial suggestion, but a quick survey of toddlers and indigenous cultures suggests an element of truth.

It's also true that while the average life expectancy is much lower, elders in such tribes tend to be more physically active than their domesticated counterparts. There are *plenty* of confounding variables here, though.

Cultures that don't rely on chairs as much as we do are much better able to get into a deep resting squat with their heels on the ground. Squatting this way can lead to greater ankle range of motion, core strength, and more.

The bottom line is indigenous cultures and more active communities certainly have us beat in *some* aspects of performance. In some cases, they even appear to possess "superhuman" abilities.

Their lifestyles change them subtly in ways that could take us months or years of adherence to a strict training regime at the gym.

---

12   This is according to acupuncturist Esther Gokhale. It's not a widely accepted view, but it certainly is interesting.

But here's the thing: someone from another culture might be equally impressed by you or me. By our ability to think abstractly with maths. By our ability to react at seventy miles per hour while driving on the motorway—and to stay focussed enough to do so for hours on end.

We can likewise point to specific jobs as creating superhuman abilities. There are obvious examples—like the amazing agility of circus performers or the incredible dexterity of concert pianists. But how about the strength and endurance of physical labourers? The juggling skills of showy bartenders?

Did you know that pro gamers have superior reaction times, visual acuity, and ability to differentiate between different shades of grey?[13] It's common knowledge that taxi drivers have larger brains owing to all the routes they need to recall.

And we've already seen how blindness can lead to echolocation and how wrestlers visualize things differently.

My argument isn't only that "natural is better." Though, I certainly think our modern environments have lost a lot of what made natural environments such good playgrounds and training areas.

Environment > Gym

If a person notices they are out of shape, feeling perhaps tired or weak, they might choose to go to the gym to fix that.

---

13   "Action Video Games Improve Vision, New Research Shows," *ScienceDaily*, March 30, 2009, https://www.sciencedaily.com/releases/2009/03/090329143326.htm.

Essentially, they are trying to make up for an entire lifetime of inactivity by training extremely hard for a few hours a week.

The ratio here is simply out of whack. If you spend eight hours a day, five days a week, sitting at work and you spend a further three hours each evening sitting on the couch, that adds up to something like sixty-one hours of sitting.

That's compared with maybe four hours at the gym.

The sitting is *by far* the bigger stimulus. And so, the adaptations caused by sitting, such as shortened hip flexors, weak glutes, hunched shoulders, tilted pelvis, strained eyes, and shallow breathing, will prevail.

To compensate, we may attempt to replace volume and frequency with intensity. Therefore, we see people attempting to squat ridiculous amounts of weight or running vast distances every week.

"Maybe if I run ten miles twice a week, I can sit as much as I like the rest of the time?"

Unsurprisingly, this often leads to injury. Especially seeing as many of these shock-and-awe style training programs lack proper balance.

This is a losing battle.

And it's why *many of us* experience lower back pain, poor overhead mobility, impaired vision, heart issues, weight gain, and even *shorter attention spans.*

Yes, this is negatively affecting your brain as well as your body.

These changes are not maladaptive, though; they are *adaptive* to the lifestyles we lead. It's a shame the lifestyles we lead are so *static*.

Your body doesn't know the difference between "training" and "not training." It doesn't know what it is "supposed" to learn from. All it knows is the environment it is being presented with.[14]

And the environment will always trump what you are doing in the gym.

We can liken this to learning a language: the best way to learn a language, reportedly, is to "immerse" yourself in it. Not to study from a book for a few hours a day but by simply travelling to another country and being constantly exposed to people speaking the local dialect.

To be naturally challenged with logical and varied goals.

The same is true when we want to improve how we move or how strong we are.

Here are several ways your everyday activities present the *far* greater stimulus.

Huge Volume

The simple fact is that when sitting, you experience a *huge volume* of stimulus. And that huge volume is always going to trump the time you spend in the gym.

We see the power of high volume in our training.

---

14   For this book, I use the term "environment" to describe not only the physical environment but also our habits and lifestyles.

While many programs advocate lifting heavy numbers and getting out of the gym as quickly as possible, others focus on high repetitions of movements.

For example, "prisoner workouts," as utilized by the likes of Mike Tyson and Charles Bronson, involve high repetitions of bodyweight squats, push-ups, and sit-ups. Mike Tyson reportedly built tree-trunk legs by performing hundreds of squats, gamified by picking cards off the ground.

This builds strength *endurance*. This is different from "max strength" in that it doesn't focus on the most you can lift in one go but instead enables you to lift heavy amounts for higher rep counts.

In the real world, strength endurance often matters more than max strength. What is the use of lifting something heavy once and placing it back down immediately? Whether wrestling, moving furniture, or performing a physical job, we need to be strong *continuously*.

This high-volume training increases max strength and strength endurance, with a preference for the latter. It also results in massive amounts of muscle growth (hypertrophy) as the body has no choice but to adapt.

High-volume training can, for example, increase the number of blood vessels supplying the muscle via angiogenesis. The repetitive use of the muscle creates a greater demand for blood and oxygen, and the body responds in kind.

Interestingly, an increase in capillarization may also lead to (or is at least correlated with) expansions of the satellite cell pool.[15] This is crucial for

15 Joshua P. Nederveen et al., "The influence of capillarization on satellite cell pool expansion and activation following exercise-induced muscle damage in healthy young men," *The Journal of Physiology* 596, no. 6 (2018):1063–1076.

hypertrophy since satellite cells fuse with muscle fibres to add myonuclei and trigger protein synthesis, adding more myonuclei in the process.

All that blood supply also means enhanced recovery. More blood and nutrients to the muscles post-exercise means a greater potential for muscle growth.

This explains why prisoners following this approach to training emerge with superhero physiques.

Another example of high-rep training comes from Tom Platz, a classic bodybuilder well-known for his incredible leg development. To accomplish this, he would reportedly perform sets of over a hundred reps on the leg-press machine. He started with light weight but eventually, he would perform huge sets with 225 pounds!

So often we admire the "one rep maximums" of athletes, but to me, this is far more impressive.

And it also explains my experiences. When I was sixteen, I started training by doing *hundreds* of push-ups every night. I'm talking five hundred repetitions or more, using a short range of motion and rapid cadence. I did something similar with pull-ups, sit-ups, and light curls (sadly, I had yet to learn the importance of not skipping leg day). This continuous time under tension and massively high volume were enough to grow some massive pecs. And to this day, I have never had any trouble gaining size around my chest and biceps.

Even cardio benefits from repeated, short bouts performed throughout the day. As neural pathways take a while to cool off post-use, so too does the cardiovascular system. Factors such as a continuously elevated heart rate and EPOC (post-exercise oxygen consumption, because acronyms can do whatever they want as long as they sound cool) mean that you gain greater overall volume this way without overtraining.

Some of these topics were discussed in my previous book, *Functional Training and Beyond*. Check it out if you want a deeper dive!

Frequency

It is not only the volume you do throughout the day. It's also the *frequency* of that training.

I'm *not* suggesting you massively ramp up your training intensity *and* volume. Not unless you want to burn out and injure yourself.

Likewise, I'm not necessarily talking about huge amounts of volume in a single set but rather spread throughout the week.

This will lead to more repetition and better learning (more on that in one sec) and may even contribute to greater *hypertrophy*.

This is especially true as we become more experienced as lifters. Protein synthesis spikes after a given workout. In a new lifter, this will return to baseline after two days. However, in a trained lifter, this returns to baseline in as little as twelve hours. Theoretically, then, training more regularly would also give you more protein synthesis and, therefore, more muscle mass.

Conflicting studies and opinions surround this, but I'm willing to go out on a limb and say it makes a lot of sense.

And this is the conclusion that YouTuber Jeff Nippard also came to when he collated this information into a video called "Full Body 5x Per Week: Why High-Frequency Training is So Effective."[16]

In one study, it was found that using the same amount of volume, athletes could gain nearly twice the amount of strength and muscle when training six times per week versus three times per week over fifteen weeks. Note, however, that this study was not published in a peer-reviewed journal.

And, of course, simply training more frequently means that you will be getting more "high quality" volume. This means you won't be as fatigued at the start of each exercise. For example: if you perform four sets of push-ups in one day, you will start the third set feeling tired. However, if you perform four sets of push-ups across two days, you will likely be coming to the third set feeling recharged after a good night's sleep.

Powerful Tendons

Higher rep training is also good for strengthening tendons. The tendons have a lesser blood supply than muscles, making them slower to respond to training. Muscle growth occurs after eight days of lifting for most new trainees, whereas it can take up to two months for the same to occur in tendons.[17]

---

16 Brad J. Schoenfeld et al., "Effects of Resistance Training Frequency on Measures of Muscle Hypertrophy: A Systematic Review and Meta-Analysis," *Sports Med,* 46, no. 11 (2016):1689–1697; Felipe Damas et al., "A review of resistance training-induced changes in skeletal muscle protein synthesis and their contributions to hypertrophy," *Sports Med.* 45, no. 6 (2015): 801–7; Cameron J. Mitchell et al., "Acute post-exercise myofibrillar protein synthesis is not correlated with resistance training-induced muscle hypertrophy in young men," *PLoS One* 9, no. 2 (2014).

17 Keitaro Kubo et al., "Time course of changes in the human Achilles tendon properties and metabolism during training and detraining in vivo," *European Journal of Applied Physiology* 112 (2011): 2679–2691.

Ben Patrick, also known as Knees Over Toes Guy, has been making waves across the fitness industry with his approach to training. In particular, and as the name suggests, he's known for rehabbing and pre-habbing the knees.

One of his best pointers for those struggling with bad knees is simply to *walk backward*. This forces the knees to move past the toes gently and naturally, placing a small amount of strain on the tendons without causing discomfort.

Ben recommends building up to a huge number of cumulative backward steps. Countless testimonials seem to suggest this works wonders.

To me, this makes perfect sense. Walking a mile backward over time presents the body with a huge *but gentle* stimulus. The stimulus is thus still powerful enough to overcome the huge volume of harmful activity that likely caused the problem in the first place.

When many of us get injured, our first instinct is to stop moving the affected area entirely. While it's important not to move through pain—that's what it's there to tell us—protecting the area from any movement simply removes any incentive for the body to prioritize healing. It also actively encourages the compensatory movement patterns that can lead to pain and further injury elsewhere.

Continuing to gently move the affected area will send blood to the area and encourage healing.

(Gentle) Movement Is Medicine

The key to effective high-volume training is to avoid extremely high intensity.

Doing hundreds of repetitions of bodyweight squats is entirely safe if done properly.[18] This method has been used by Indian wrestlers, such as the legendary Gama, for centuries.

However, doing hundreds of repetitions of *heavy back squats* is less advisable.

Pavel Tsatsouline tells the story of weightlifter Vasily Alexeev. Alexeev had back pain and could not perform deadlifts. Instead, he would use slow repetitions of back hypers using a relatively light forty to sixty kilos and lots of volume.

These slow repetitions, as it happens, have many of the same benefits as super high reps. That is to say that the "time under tension" and the total volume are drastically increased. However, the intensity remains manageable.

A lot of people would struggle to recover if they ran ten miles every day. However, those same people would likely be in excellent health if they walked the same distance!

This is why authors like Ben Greenfield recommend running at significantly lower intensities than the prevalent "black hole" training[19] performed under the lactate threshold.[20]

---

18 No, you don't need to worry about "repetitive strain," and we'll get to why and how to avoid this in the next chapter.

19 This is the kind of running most of us gravitate toward when trying to "feel an effect." We run fast enough to make it extremely difficult rather than taking a much slower, more gentle job.

20 Ben Greenfield, *Beyond Training: Mastering Endurance, Health & Life* (New York: Victory Belt, 2018).

This kind of high-volume, low-intensity activity is the kind of stimulus our everyday activities provide.

Looked at in this way, sitting *is* training. So is sawing if that's your job. So is lifting your kid in and out of the cot.

And the effect might be *more* profound than what you're doing in the gym.

The problem is that a lot of that stimulus is not good for us.

Greasing the Groove

High volume, low intensity is also optimal when it comes to learning.

This is exemplified by another concept described by Pavel Tsatsouline. "Greasing the groove" is the process of repeating a certain activity throughout the day.

A popular example is keeping a pull-up bar in the doorway and performing pull-ups every time you go through.

This strengthens the "skill component" of a movement. While the physical size and strength of your muscle plays a role in your power output, your efficiency in movement is arguably just as, if not *more* important.

Movement patterns that you perform are effectively saved in the brain as "engrams." The series of neurons necessary to perform the movement are connected via synapses, and these connections become more efficient with every repetition. The axon gets better insulated by myelination and the "incorrect" connections are culled.

Like sawing at a tree and making the groove deeper and deeper with each stroke.

Were you to take a glimpse at the brain of a pro athlete versus an amateur, the athlete's brain would show a far more defined series of connections, whereas the amateur would have a lot more "noise." Over time, the correct path is reinforced until there is far less deviation from the "ideal" movement.

On a physical level, this results in the more efficient firing of motor units within the muscle (which is to say that you get better at calling upon the strength in the muscle) and better coordination of the correct *groups* of muscles together. The muscles you want to activate work in tandem while the antagonists become more relaxed.

If you repeat the movement throughout the day, you're able to reinforce that movement pattern repeatedly, without causing damage or fatigue in the muscle.

So, if you sew for a living, you will become extremely efficient and dextrous at doing that. There will be minimal wasted energy.

If you also squat at the gym, you probably practiced that movement *far less* than the sewing!

Spaced Learning

What often gets overlooked here is the benefit of "spaced learning." Spaced learning is a strategy that breaks a single learning "session" into multiple, smaller blocks. Rather than sitting down to revise for a test for two hours straight, you might instead have four half-hour blocks.

Studies show that this approach can significantly enhance learning outcomes.[21] Why is this?

For one, spacing out learning simply prevents fatigue and loss of focus. A two-hour learning session is intense. Half an hour is far more appealing for most of us. This means you're likely to be more focussed and have a more productive total learning experience.

This can go double for a workout where physical fatigue is a real challenge!

What's more is that any learning session will incur a "cool-off period" of sorts. After you have memorized a subject, the neurons and nerves will remain somewhat more active thanks to short-term plasticity, a.k.a. dynamical synapses. This makes it easier to trigger them again.

We can even experience this subjectively—as you will find, you're likely to absent-mindedly rehearse or think about what you just learned.

By employing a distributed practice strategy, you gain *multiple* cool-off periods.

This also makes the *start* of each learning block slightly more difficult because you are retrieving those memories from "cold." This may help you to practice calling upon information with no prep time. And fittingly, this is also how we retrieve and use information in the real world.

---

21   Paul Kelley and Terry Whatson, "Making long-term memories in minutes: a spaced learning pattern from memory research in education," *Front Hum Neuroscience* 7 (2013): 589.

Learning also increases several neurotrophic compounds that enhance brain plasticity: such as BDNF (brain-derived neurotrophic factor), dopamine, acetylcholine, and nerve growth factor. By spiking these neurotransmitters, you put your brain into a state of heightened learning. By doing it multiple times throughout the day, you benefit from *multiple* spikes in plasticity.

This also occurs in the rest of the body. Training spikes hormones like testosterone increases protein synthesis, thus increasing the metabolism to burn more fat.

Train multiple times per day, and you spike all these things multiple times per day, as well.

Contextual Interference

I am describing the benefits of spaced learning because it is once again something that occurs naturally when you let the environment train you.

You're such a great sitting machine because you not only sit with massive volume but you also sit multiple times per day.

Any action you must frequently repeat, without even thinking, will get seared indelibly into your grey matter.

But our lifestyles don't only impact us through spaced learning. They also have the benefit of "contextual interference."

The contextual interference effect shows us that mixing and matching different movements in a single session will impact the way we learn those movements.

When you go to the gym to train, you will normally have a list of exercises to perform. You will then perform each exercise for a set number of repetitions in a row. You might do three-by-ten bicep curls, for example. Or three-by-four heavy barbell squats.

Conversely, when moving out in the real world, we will rarely perform the same movement repeatedly. The same goes for sports. Or manual labour.

When cleaning the kitchen, you will walk, bend, lift, scrub, carry, and more. All out of sequence.

A footballer will sprint, jog, walk, dribble, kick, jump, then pretend to be injured. All out of sequence.

So, if you want to train someone to shoot a hoop in basketball or netball, should you get them to stand in one spot and train the shot over and over again? And then should they have a separate "block" of cardio? A separate block of dribbling?

Or do you mix those things up?

According to the studies, mixing the training so multiple skills are challenged out of sequence will impair performance during practice. However, this will also translate to *greater* performance and retention *post* training.[22]

Theoretically, this makes it harder to apply what we are training in the gym to our lives *outside* the gym. And it means that all those habits we learn passively are much more likely to stick.

---

22 João Barrieros et al., "The contextual interference effect in applied settings," *Eur Phys Educ Rev* 13, no. 2 (2007): 195–208.

Repetition without Repetition

But perhaps the real secret sauce here is variety. Repetition *without* repetition.

What we consider "training" is often comprised of blocks of precise repetitious movements.

But the natural environment that shapes us so effortlessly is categorically *not* that. There are never two motions exactly alike.

By moving naturally through a wild environment, you *automatically* provide your body with various stimuli.

Imagine lifting a log versus lifting a heavy weight. When lifting a rock, you are forced to grip the rock, as you can't simply wrap your hands around the bar.

Because the rock will likely be asymmetrical, you will need to brace your core on one side, engaging the oft-overlooked quadratus lumborum, multifidus muscles, and obliques to stabilize. You'll need to plant yourself on the ground so as not to fall over, and you'll need to push with different amounts of force through each side of your upper body.

And because the ground is uneven and the terrain varied, you'll also need to listen to proprioceptive feedback from your feet as you balance through your ankles and feet.

The same thing happens when you climb a tree or a cliff. Perform a pull-up from a bar and you'll be performing the same linear movement across a straight bar, over and over.

And, of course, the same thing happens every time you lift a spoon full of cereal: the weight changes, and you likely change position as you talk to your daughter about *Paw Patrol*.

The same thing happens every time you lift the pram into the boot of your car. Every time you put up a tent.

Perform the *same* exercise on a tree branch and it will be different every time. Now your grip will be challenged by different width branches. Some parts will be slippery, too. You may also find that one hand is higher than the other or that the branch bends and has some give.

If you now also change the *intention* of the pull-up—such that you're climbing the tree rather than repeating the movement—then you'll also be varying your tempo, positions, and more. Sometimes, you'll pull yourself up and to the left. Sometimes, you'll need to hang from one arm while you find another place to hang with the other. Sometimes, you'll need to explode upwards to reach a higher rung. Your technique *and* cadence will be varied.

Trail running has the same benefit as running. When you trail run, your ankles, feet, and knees are under increased stress due to the uneven surface. This provides more proprioceptive feedback, training the body to better balance and stabilize, and strengthens those tendons. In one study, it was found that habitual barefoot running could improve sprint times in children: by decreasing ground-contact time and increasing jump height.[23]

The varied, chaotic stimulus that moving and working outdoors offers builds *much* more useful and transferrable strength versus performing the same few lifts with a straight bar. Military pressing might build bigger

---

23 Jun Mizushima et al., "Long-term effects of school barefoot running program on sprinting biomechanics in children: A case-control study," *Gait & Posture* 83 (2021): 9–14.

shoulders and help you lift more at the gym, but you won't learn to stabilize your core in the same way, and your grip will lack.

Should someone need to lift furniture or grapple a constantly moving opponent, the log press will provide better preparation.

How Log Press Makes You Bulletproof

What's more is that the log press, trail running, and tree climbing will all make you more resilient to injury.

A quick look around YouTube fitness will show you that most people who go to the gym are afraid of their own shadow. Push-ups are dangerous if performed with elbows flared. Flexion in the spine during a deadlift is essentially a one-way ticket to the hospital. Oh, and don't let your knees pass your toes.

No, I don't know how you will get down the stairs... That's your problem.

In fact, you know what? Don't even look at a weight until you've had at least five years of being shouted at by strangers on the internet. It's too dangerous!

Meanwhile, my three-year-old daughter leaps off the sofa that's twice her height and lands on her *knees* without blinking.

I'm not suggesting you do the latter, but I *am* demonstrating how fragile we've become. And the reason is that we've avoided all movement except for a few precise movement patterns.

This is one of the central concepts behind the movement training culture, which Tom Myers discusses in his book, *Anatomy Trains*. Tom Myer explains that constantly training with the same linear vectors will strengthen only particular parts of the fascia, while areas right next to those go untrained. These areas may thus become tight and inflexible or simply weak and prone to injury.

Even walking on natural terrain provides a far richer experience than walking on flat ground, especially if you vary your route and wear a thinner-soled shoe with minimal heel drop.

If you train yourself only in a few linear positions, you'll be strong in those positions and nowhere else.

Degrees of Freedom and Athletic Performance

Moreover, our nervous system also benefits greatly from the varied movement offered by the natural environment.

This is well-demonstrated by a problem known as the "degrees of freedom problem," postulated by Nicolai Bernstein. This thought experiment highlights the significant challenge the body faces in simply moving around. Because, even to do the simplest thing, there are *countless* options and available methods.

Want to pick up a sock? How does your body unconsciously decide which leg to put forward, how far to twist, at which point to hinge, and at which point to bend the back?

This is possible, of course, thanks to the nervous system. According to dynamical systems theory, movement is narrowed down by constraints, which include the goal, the environment, and the organism. That is to say that every movement must organize itself around these three factors. And thus, every movement will be different every time.

Even seemingly "linear" movements like the bench press will still vary based on the precise position of your hands, how fatigued you are from the previous day, and the precise amount of momentum carried over from the last set.

And, of course, something like swinging a baseball bat will be drastically different based on the terrain, footwear, speed of the incoming ball, and more.

From there, Bernstein described how certain body parts might be "frozen" to reduce the number of moving parts. In other words: we keep one part of the body static so that we have less to consider while unpredictably moving through space. Others might be "coupled" such that the trajectory of the wrist mirrors that of the elbow.[24]

Freezing body parts is not the most efficient way to move the body, as it results in reduced adaptability. Thus, as the practitioner masters their technique, they will begin "freeing" body parts.

Learning the tornado kick from my friend Grant last week, I noticed this in effect. It was harder to move gracefully because my torso was rigid as I spun in the air. Thing is, that was the only way to prevent me from crash landing!

---

24 Bernstein suggested that this might occur in a specific order: proximal to distal—starting from the trunk and radiating out to the extremities.

A few studies have addressed to what degree this "freezing and freeing" accurately describes the learning process when acquiring new skills. In short, this gets deep.

But the point is that it appears the body needs to be given variety to *truly* master a movement. In one study,[25] for example, it was shown that having "more variability in practice conditions" could help baseball batters to better solve coordination challenges and, thus, improve performance.

Whereas many gym rats worship at the altar of "perfect repetition," the reality may be different. To be a truly free mover, we need dynamic challenges.

We need analogue training, not binary!

This is adaptive training. This is being trained almost by osmosis, through variety, volume, and frequency rather than short bouts of intense exercise.

So, what am I proposing here?

How might we get to a place where our environment can train us in a positive manner?

Well, you'll have to keep reading the next chapters, won't you?

25   Rob Gray, "Changes in Movement Coordination Associated with Skill Acquisition in Baseball Batting: Freezing/Freeing Degrees of Freedom and Functional Variability," *Front Psychol* 11 (2020): 1295.

Chapter 3

CREATING THE IDEAL, STIMULATING ENVIRONMENT

There *are* some practical ways to immediately implement everything we've learned into our training.

For example, you might decide to start training with lighter weights and high repetition. Now, I don't want to encourage throwing out any babies with any bathwater here.

Of course, there are benefits to high-intensity training. There is undoubtedly a time and place for lifting heavy stuff or sprinting.

But what I *would* recommend is *also* including high-repetition work. For example, you might perform your heavy bench presses during your workout but end with high-rep push-ups as a finisher. This would flood the area with blood and stimulate further growth following your training.

This way, we bring one of the natural benefits of adaptive training to our workouts while still doing everything we're used to.

That's the tip of the iceberg, of course.

Greasing the Groove

If you want to learn a skill more rapidly, you should employ the strategy of greasing the groove. Practice those skills throughout the day, being mindful not to overly tax the body each time. Want to learn to handstand? Try holding a handstand a couple of times a day without reaching fatigue and you'll learn much faster.

Failing this, if you have any skill-based component of your regular workouts, I recommend spacing them out throughout the session. For example, if you hit the gym for an hour, you could practice the handstand at the start of the session, in the middle, and at the end (fatigue allowing, of course).

Vector Sets

This is where things get more interesting.

I'd also recommend that you *consider* mixing up your reps. The obsession most gym-goers have with robotically repeating precisely prescribed movements is strange.

When you step back and think about it…

"Don't mind me! I'm just going to stand here and pick up and put down this weight in the same way for a while."

"How long?"

"Maybe, like, a minute and a half?"

"Okay."

"Then again, twice more."

"Righto."

Instead of performing a hundred push-ups, why not alternate each repetition between push-ups, Hindu push-ups, clapping push-ups, slow push-ups, knuckle push-ups, archer push-ups, one-armed push-ups, and whatever other variation you fancy?

I call these **Vector Sets**.

(Again, this doesn't have to completely replace your normal training. It's a protocol to introduce if you want to shake things up and perhaps bust through some plateaus.)

The key is that the movements should target *broadly* the same muscles. They should be "similar but different."

This would not only help you benefit from contextual interference but also keep the exercise *far* more interesting and engaging. This would make it more implicitly motivating, making you more likely to *want* to perform the exercise. And it would simultaneously up the challenge quite significantly.

You may also find that Vector Sets leave you feeling sorer and more challenged than regular sets. This is because you can no longer rely on momentum, rhythm, or repetition. Every movement requires you to "reset" as it were, to shift your centre of gravity slightly and to engage slightly different parts of the body.

You also need to concentrate on the transition *between* the movements.

Going from a push-up to a one-armed push-up, for example, means shifting your gravity over one hand and probably widening your feet.

But we're *still* focussing on specific areas enough to create muscle damage, metabolic stress—all that good stuff that leads to growth.[26]

Applying Vector Sets in Your Workouts

The same process can be applied to any exercise, pretty much. Used to doing curl after curl? How about alternating between curls, hammer curls, slow curls, pronated grip curls, Zottman curls, and drag curls?

Look up these movements if that was a bunch of gibberish to you.

The point is there is little reason to perform three sets of ten repetitions of the same movement three times a week. This *isn't* how we move in the real world. If we want to emulate the environment we're preparing for, we need to include variety and unpredictability in our training.

Bruce Lee said he didn't fear the man who had practiced a thousand different kicks. Rather, he feared the man who had practiced one kick a thousand times.

There is definite truth to this.

But I think *I* would most fear the man who had practiced one kick a thousand different ways!

Note that Vector Sets should also include varied tempos. For example: you might perform your explosive push-ups then switch to an isometric

---

26   And which we'll be tackling in an upcoming section.

hold or slow, quasi-isometric push-up before returning to fast knuckle push-ups or a lizard crawl.

The importance of varying cadence during Vector Sets will become apparent later in this book.

Learning vs. Training

Is this the optimal way to continuously get better at those movements? Not at all. But the point of sharpening an axe is not to get better at sharpening an axe; it's to *make a sharper axe*.

I highly recommend when you are initially learning a movement, you keep the variables as constant as possible to hone your technique. *But*, once mastered, start varying the precise conditions to keep yourself engaged and challenged and to prepare to use that movement the way it would be used.

Even if you don't want to go as far as to utilize different tempos and movement patterns within a single set, you can still get a much wider variety by using different variations of the same exercise in each set.

For example: set one might be a squat. Set two might be a squat with a wider stance. Set three might be an explosive jumping squat.

We can call these **Quasi-Vector Sets**.

Same muscle groups, same muscle damage, greater stimulation, and better transfer to real-world situations.

Just Go Outside!

Want to incorporate some of the benefits of being outdoors into
your training?

Then, uh, be outdoors!

Being outside means you benefit from sun exposure, fresh air, and
natural views, but it *also* provides your body with a unique stimulus
that it can't get from the gym. And that stimulus is perfect for building
stronger, more supple, and flexible bodies. The alternative is to be
extremely strong in certain areas and weak in others while also being
tight and immobile. Can you see how that might lead to injury?

The solution traditionally offered by many coaches is to make sure you
don't forget the smaller muscles that can lead to imbalances and injuries
when overlooked.

This is why we are prescribed movements like the face pull to train the
rotator cuffs and prevent shoulder injury. Reverse hypers can help to
ease back pain. An overhand grip on the barbell during grips can fend off
tennis elbow. Tibialis raises can prevent shin splints. The list goes on.

The problem is that this can be a little reductionist in its approach. And
you risk ending up with a *huge* list of prehab exercises to perform that
are all boring and time-consuming. Chances are you're still going to
miss a lot.

And this is where the natural environment, or at least varied, natural
movement, offers the perfect solution. By providing unlimited, varying
stimuli for the body, simply moving and training outside can strengthen
all these varied areas almost by osmosis.

It treats the body as a black box. Instead of trying to understand every tendon and joint and train them equally, we move naturally with widely varied movement and let it take care of itself. Nothing pulls ahead as being disproportionately trained as a result.

For example: to train the tibialis anterior, a muscle responsible for raising the toes upwards (dorsiflexion) that also helps handle impacts during a jump or sprint, we simply need to swim or run uphill.

Want to strengthen the rotator cuff muscles? Rock climbing will do that. Especially if you are *traversing*. Here, you climb horizontally across a wall, requiring you to constantly pull yourself in toward the wall.

I call this the "Black Box Approach to Training." Here, we are acknowledging and accepting our limitations in understanding the human body and instead relying on the ready-made tool the body evolved to interface with: the environment.

Humans: The Natural Climbers

"Hang on!" You might be saying, somewhat pun-ishly.

"Is climbing that natural a movement? Is this how we would have developed our rotator cuffs in the wild?"

"Didn't we *descend* from the trees?"

Well, yes. And yes, climbing *and* some activities, such as throwing, would have helped develop the rotator cuffs.

There is a lot of evidence for climbing as a natural human endeavour, rather than the mostly white-middle-class hobby it has more recently been viewed as.

While many credit Parry Haskett Smith as the "father of rock climbing," having popularized it as a pastime in 1886, it dates back much further.

Like, duh! If there be rocks, people are gunsta' climb them!

For starters, there is now plenty of prehistoric evidence of early man climbing. Cave paintings show ropes used for climbing dating back around 45,000 years.

Climbing has also served as an important part of many cultures. The Nepalese Sherpa are well-known for their mountaineering. Ancient Puebloans once lived inside cliff dwellings that could only be accessed by climbing the mesas. The Igorot tribe in the Northern Philippines bury their dead in coffins that hang from vertical cliff faces.

Then there are China's Miao people, also known as "Spider Men," who free solo to access traditional herbs.

And there are the Twa, whom we've already met.

The point is that climbing is a birth right we all share and one that has helped to shape our bodies.

Wild Training, in Comfort

So, what am I suggesting you do here?

Firstly: train outdoors where possible. Make like Tarzan!

Become *half wild*.

I will regularly train outside, whether at a nature reserve, a park, or open countryside. This started during lockdown, especially because I needed somewhere other than my garden to film for my YouTube channel. But the huge advantages soon made themselves clear.

Rather than heading to your local gym, set off for a beauty spot and perform your workout there.

How can you train without equipment? Well, first, who said anything about not having equipment?

But to answer the question: you *can* always prefer bodyweight exercises for most of your workouts. There are plenty of resources online teaching bodyweight training. All we're going to do is do that same thing somewhere pretty.

Push-ups and handstands on the grass, pull-ups and front levers from tree branches, pistol squats on a park bench—it's simple.

Of course, you *will* progress slightly more slowly when it comes to those advanced calisthenics skills because the environment will make them harder (I'm talking planche, front lever, etc.). *But* you will build more useful, real-world strength, provide the brain with greater stimulus, and potentially prevent injury. All that good stuff we've talked about.

While you're at it, why not throw in some resistance training with what you have available?

A great move is finding a felled tree branch and performing landmine presses. Or perform some overhead presses with a log. Or traverse around a tree. You can even do some swimming for a cardio finisher. Or a hill sprint. Which is brilliant for tons of reasons.

There are countless options.

Gym bros will scoff and ask how you can see meaningful progression without progressive overload or measuring your precise weights.

Again, though, we're not interested in progressing specific lifts for their own sake! As long as you regularly push yourself close to failure, you will elicit a positive change in your body.

Numbers Don't Matter

In fact, this is something that truly confuses me: why do some people seem to believe you can only improve if you can measure that improvement? And why do you need numbers to tell you if you've gone to failure or not? Or putting in meaningful effort?

Far more important than the number of lbs or kg on your barbell is your RPE (Rate of Perceived Effort). That's a number that works wherever you are in the world.

And hey, if you miss seeing those numbers go up, return to the same logs and try and increase your rep count. If you used to be able to do ten presses of that log and now you can do eleven, you know you're improving. *Or* throw in a few traditional gym workouts alongside your more varied training style.

Of course, when it comes to calisthenics, you can simply progress as you normally would. Just expect that progress to be a little less linear.

That's a good thing.

Tools with Many Vectors

Another option is to train in your usual environment while using *tools* that naturally offer more vectors of resistance and more variation.

For example, rather than performing the clean and press with a barbell, you could do the same thing with two kettlebells.[27] Or with a sandbag.[28] Or a backpack, even!

The kettlebells are great because they have an offset centre of gravity, which means they'll shift and move as you lift them. You need to deal not only with the weight's resistance but also the significant momentum and balance challenge.

Sandbags take this one step further: here the weight shifts *within* the sandbag, meaning that no two lifts are remotely identical. This is what we call "unaccommodating resistance." It's the same kind of resistance you'd deal with when lifting a person or even a shopping bag.

---

27 Large iron balls with handles sticking out the top.
28 Big heavy bags full of sand or something else.

Variety Is the Spice of Life

And, of course, you can get many of these same benefits by using more variety in your workouts. The Vector Sets we discussed earlier can be highly beneficial because each movement is different. You can likewise use the recently popular "flows" or hybrid exercises. These are sequences of movements performed for reps. Flows are typically sequences of three or four movements, whereas hybrid exercises are two to three exercises combined.

For example, you might perform a one-armed kettlebell swing to a snatch while stepping back into a backward lunge. You then stand up, swing, swap arms, and repeat.

Alternatively, a burpee is another hybrid exercise as it incorporates both a push-up and a squat jump. Look up the devil press or man-maker for slightly more complex combos.

In all these scenarios, you are not only performing a range of movements and training more vectors, but you're also training the positions *between* those movements and handling the momentum and changing angles as you do.

The simplest expression of this concept, though, is simply to use a greater variety of movements in your training.

The Barefoot Advantage

Another "tool" for making *any* training and *any* activity much more "natural" is the barefoot shoe. These are shoes designed to more closely resemble the experience of being barefoot.

I have discussed this in my previous book and countless articles on my site, so I won't go into it in detail here... *But* because I'm a terrible bore, I *will* recap some of the key benefits.

Removing your shoes instantly alters your natural running and walking gait for the better. When running, you will now favour landing on the ball of your foot. This is the padded part of the foot, after all. This means you won't strike the ground with your leg out in front of your knee extended (an invitation for knee problems). Instead, your foot lands underneath your centre of gravity, allowing your ankle, knee, and hip to flex and fully absorb the impact of the landing.

This also allows the toes to splay and better contour to the ground (preventing twisted ankles) and to push off the ground, strengthening the toe muscles such as the flexor hallucis longus and flexor digitorum longus.

Look at someone who has transitioned to a barefoot lifestyle or just "minimal footwear," and you will see that they have naturally more splayed-out toes. This is how our toes *should* look. Again, our natural lifestyles have imposed a profound and negative physical change upon us.

A raised heel puts the foot into permanent plantar flexion, preventing us from properly pushing off the ground to generate maximum force. This also puts the calf into a permanently shortened and tightened position, contributing to the fact that many of us cannot squat *or* touch our toes.

Then there is the sheer amount of proprioception—information from your body—you lose when you run on a thick sole. Try balancing along a log barefoot and it's an entirely different experience, as you can feel the bark underneath you and how your balance shifts.

It's also this proprioception that allows our unconscious gait to perform optimally. Author James Earls explains in his book *Born to Walk* how in-built reflexes help us to walk while expending the smallest amount of energy.

For example, when your heel touches the ground, you have a *natural* reflex to plantar flex. This is triggered by mechanoreceptors (more on these later) that sense changes in the length and tension of the plantar fascia. Similarly, when the pressure is relieved, reflexes kick in to automatically dorsiflex the foot: raising it above potential obstacles to prevent us from tripping.

Stimulate the bottom of the foot and you will naturally grip with your toes. This "plantar reflex" is designed to help us grip onto the ground and thus not fall over.

Now imagine the huge impact that wearing shoes will have on this. When your heel is so cushioned, those signals are significantly blunted.

And over time, we can lose our ability to sense these things *at all*.

Is it a wonder so many elderly people injure themselves by falling down the stairs? Shuffling, as they are, in thick slippers?[29] After years of neglecting the natural proprioception of their feet?

Dividing Workouts

For this book and the goals we've outlined and discussed thus far, I recommend training with whole-body workouts or at least a Push, Pull,

---

29 That shuffling, FYI, is due to a lack of dorsiflexion, either because of a weak anterior tibialis or a lack of proper signalling.

Legs split. The latter means you are training all pushing movements, then all pulling movements, then the legs. I also like the Push, Pull, Legs, Full Body setup.

If we're aiming to emulate how the environment *naturally* shapes us, then we should involve a high level of frequency. This also makes up for a relatively lower intensity.

This increase in frequency can stimulate more growth and by "hitting biceps" three times per week, you'll see faster and greater changes.

But that doesn't have to mean you perform biceps three times a week. If the biceps are the prime movers of a given exercise, a vast range of different movements will be just as effective.

So, for example, you could perform bicep curls on Monday, chin ups on Tuesday, and cheat curls on Thursday.

Instead of repeating hamstring curls multiple times per week, why not perform hamstring curls, Nordic curls, and Romanian deadlifts? Again, you'll get far more benefits and all the same hypertrophy and strength gains. Again, you can look up these moves, but that's not the point. The point is: there's no reason to do the same movements three times per week.

This way, you also get all those nice "secondary benefits" that each exercise brings. For example, you'll strengthen your lower back with the RDLs and improve your deadlift.

Or why not perform one of each movement instead of three sets of anything? There are those quasi-Vector Sets, again. This requires more work and understanding—you need to know which muscle groups each movement targets and how to make sure you feel the benefits in the right place. But with the right program/coach/research, this is doable.

High Frequency & Volume

The other thing to consider when looking at how we can emulate the qualities of natural training is frequency.

The Twa pigmy tribe, with their amazing climbing abilities, can do what they do because they started climbing at a young age. It's also because they have that great balance of "variety and consistency" that I've been talking about.

But it's *also* because they climb so regularly. And this is a huge deal when it comes to the power of the environment to shape your body.

So, am I suggesting you bench press forty reps a day, every day, to become an amazing powerlifter?

Not exactly. I have a few tricks for achieving this end, which I have kindly shared in the next chapter.

I'll see you there.

Man, I think I've gotten cheesier since becoming a dad.

Chapter 4

TRAINING THROUGHOUT THE DAY–NEVER STOP TRAINING!

The other way we can tap into the incredible adaptive powers of the human body when training is by exposing ourselves sporadically to "training" stimuli throughout the day.

In our natural environment, we would not have spent hours sitting in one position only to torch ourselves with pull-ups on a tree branch. I feel we've established this well at this point.

Sure, we would have rested from time to time. But we would also have walked a lot, hunted, fought, climbed, carried, and more. This wasn't structured; it was dictated by our needs and the whims of the environment.

Thus, the "main" stimulus required mobility, strength, endurance, and agility.

In other words, rather than one long, intense workout, we would have had repeated bouts of moderate exercise.

We can do the same thing.

Farmer Strength

If we combine these ingredients, we get what some refer to as "farmer strength." Farmer strength is the kind of strength often displayed by farmers, often associated with manual labourers.

You might also have heard people talk about "dad strength" or "mum strength." Many of us remember the vice-like grip our dads had when they grabbed our wrists.

That was just our perception as a little dude or dudette, right?

Maybe not.

As a dad, I am constantly active. Getting the kids ready for the day is like wrestling octopuses.[30] Or perhaps colossal squids.

Krakens.

I often have to carry both my three-year-old (she's nearly four) and my seven-month-old up the stairs. They have a combined weight of twenty-three kilograms. And talk about unaccommodating resistance!

When I get back from the office (a.k.a. The Biolab), my daughter likes to play a game called "playground." Here, I have to use my body to recreate various items at the playground. She climbs me like a climbing frame. I perform kettlebell swings with her to simulate the swing. I swing her round like a roundabout. And I do pike pulses with her hanging onto my feet to be the see-saw.

This is one of our more relaxing games.

---

30 Yes, this is the correct plural!

Combine this with all the chores I now need to do, like painting the ceiling two days ago, carrying the broken fence into the front garden the other day, or tidying the living room every night. I'm never still for long.

This type of movement has all the varied vectors, grip challenge, and more that makes for the perfect stimulus. The result is that dads and mums are adapted to exert moderate strength in a wide range of positions for long periods.

My wife has pretty decent biceps right now.

This is considerably *more* true for farmers, labourers, and others. Hence "farmer strength."

They have higher intensity during their activities. And they don't get to escape to "work" for eight hours a day.

Manual work, like digging a hole, means being highly physical for hours at a time with little breaks. This creates amazing strength and endurance.

All this physicality is performed in a manner that has minimal repetition and lots of unpredictability. When lifting something heavy from the floor at an awkward angle, the labourer must use their grip strength while bracing their core to stabilize themselves and still exert power through the limbs.

Digging a hole means training the often-neglected rotational strength in the transverse plane: working the obliques and hips. At the same time, the grip experiences a significant challenge as the dirt sits at the end of a long lever, increasing the subjective resistance.

And because the hole gets deeper with each load, the precise angle and position will change with *every* repetition.

Modular Training

Another way to emulate this more natural style of movement and training that hasn't been fully addressed is to train multiple times per day, rather than just once.

As gym-goers, we tend to take instruction at face value. We assume there is a good reason for what we are advised to do and don't question it.

For example: most of us naturally train with three sets of a single exercise. It doesn't help that studies show that three sets provide the greatest stimulus for growth.

But those studies don't ask what happens when you use three *similar but different* exercises. And so, many of us are afraid to try it.

Similarly, I *for years* assumed that breaking my workouts into smaller chunks would damage my gains. Heck, I was afraid to spend too long talking to other gym patrons in case I "lost my pump."

(Also, because I'm an awkward person.)

But, as it happens, nothing could be further from the truth.

(Not the part about being awkward; that's true.)

Here's what happens when you take a one-hour workout and break it into three twenty-minute workouts or two thirty-minute workouts:

- Each workout starts fresh, meaning you have more energy to go harder on those first exercises.

- If you incorporate similar movements, you benefit from the "greasing the groove" effect and "spaced learning." This can apply even to motor unit recruitment (theoretically), so the movements don't need to be identical.

- You spike your heart rate two or three times during the day rather than just once because it takes a while for the blood to slow.

- You flood the muscles with blood multiple times per day.

- You spike protein synthesis multiple times per day. In trained individuals, protein synthesis takes about twelve hours to return to baseline; this is *not* a binary but a spectrum.

In short, rather than compromising your gains, this training style *enhances* them. Significantly.

This is something I've experienced myself on multiple occasions. It's something I've seen when training others. My friend Simon got *huge* by training once in the morning and once in the evening.

And some studies back it up, too.[31] In fact, evidence suggests that this can benefit everything from fat loss to protein synthesis to strength gains and more!

Is It Practical to Break Up Workouts?

I always wanted to try this because it works better with my unusual routine. For me, it can be hard to find a whole hour to train. Especially if that needs to incorporate a commute to the gym and a change of clothes.

---

31 Daniel A Corrêa et al., "Twice-daily sessions result in a greater muscle strength and a similar muscle hypertrophy compared to once-daily sessions in resistance-training men," *J Sports Med Phys Fitness* 62, no. 3 (2022): 324–336; Andrew J.R. Cochran et al., "Manipulating Carbohydrate Availability Between Twice-Daily Sessions of High-Intensity Interval Training Over 2 Weeks Improves Time-Trial Performance," *Int Journ Sport Nut Exerc Metab* 25, no. 5 (2014): 463–470; Victoria Amorim Andrade-Souza et al., "Exercise twice-a-day potentiates markers of mitochondrial biogenesis in men," *The FASEB Journal* 34, no. 1 (2019): 1602–1619.

I barely have enough time to finish my work as it is, so I can't easily take time out of my working day. I wake up at six or seven in the morning and don't get time to work until eight thirty or nine o'clock on account of getting the kids ready.

And when I finish work at four thirty or five o'clock, I want to come home to *be* with my children.

I *can* manage thirty minutes at the start of the day and thirty minutes before bed. And maybe an additional ten minutes of curls or handstand practice at the office.

(My office is…*different*.)

But I also recognize that this style of training is not for everyone. Other people might find it easier to dedicate a block of time to their training and leave it at that.

And there are some unique challenges to training multiple times per day. Perhaps the one that comes up most often when I talk about this is *sweat*. Multiple workouts mean multiple showers, right? And what about warm-ups and cool-downs? If you do three workouts, you're looking at three warm-ups of ten minutes each, right? So, you're spending nearly thirty minutes just warming up?

A lot of this will be subjective and will depend on your circumstances, goals, and…well, *sweatiness*, I guess.

Genetically, some people need more time to warm up than others. This may be due to differing levels of resting *adrenaline*.

But here are some points to consider:

The Challenge of Warming Up

A warm-up genuinely needn't take more than a few minutes. Get the blood flowing with some light cardio, then practice unweighted versions of the movements you'll be using. That said, individual differences apply here, and your age and other factors will likely impact how much of a warm-up you need.

With that said, having trained previously during the day should mean you're already a little warmer for the second workout. Theoretically, most people can utilize a shorter workout the second and third times they train. More on this in a moment.

Also consider that warming up shouldn't be viewed as a waste of time. Use warm-ups that actively benefit your training in their own way. Not all your training should consist of heavy lifts or intense running; the rest can be used as a gentle warm-up. I might do a little bag work and focus on skills to get the blood circulating. Then I might do some hand balancing (more of a skill-based challenge than a strength challenge). Or perhaps I'll do some ATG split squats (relatively light) or hip thrusts. These aren't a waste of time but are legitimate parts of the workout that *happen* to warm me up in a safe way.

Time

As mentioned, time can be an issue, depending on who you are and how your routine works.

One solution, I find, is to compromise by having a "main workout" and "peripheral" workouts. If I'm pushed for time but still manage to get to the gym/outdoors, I will get as much done during that time as I can. I'll also aim to prioritize anything that *can't* be done at home or the office.

This way, I can do those missing extra bits later. For example: I might do pull-ups, deadlifts, and rows at the gym and then, later that night, come home to do some face pulls using bands.

This also illustrates the importance of having multiple places to work out. I personally train:

- At the gym
- At home in the living room
- In my office (BIOLAB)
- In the garden
- In parks and fields

To do this, I keep a few dumbbells and a set of dip bars in the office. My living room has a big open space in the middle for bodyweight training (I also have two small wooden parallettes).

The garden has a pull-up bar mounted to the wall with a rope hanging from it and an eyelet for a heavy bag (in the shed). I keep a medicine ball and a couple of other things in my boot.

And I *always* have resistance bands in my pocket/shoulder bag.

With these tools, I can get a workout in wherever I go!

Sweat

This is one of the biggest challenges, in all honesty. Training for fifteen minutes can still make you sweaty on a hot day, leading to embarrassment at the office or even skin issues.

There's no easy answer to this; you'll need to find what works for you.

A few tips, though:

- If you know you won't have a chance to shower, try to stick to lighter training options
- Find somewhere with good air conditioning/a fan
- Take your top off, where appropriate
- Keep a carrier bag on you with a spare change of clothes and deodorant
- In most cases, splashing water under your armpits, spraying deodorant, and changing your top should be enough to address any smells.

That said, for short workouts, it is less of an issue.

Something you can do is to perform a single Vector Set to failure. This logically leads to the question, "How small can we go?" Well, according to Mike Mentzer, the single factor that truly matters in any given workout is that you "[get] to a point where you are forced to utilize 100 percent of your momentary ability."

We can achieve this with a single set, so long as the focus remains on one group of muscles, i.e., a Vector Set performed to failure.

Repeat that same Vector Set multiple times throughout the day for a huge amount of variation, spaced repetition, greasing the groove, and frequency.

And you shouldn't sweat all that much.

Overtraining

Another concern for many people is overtraining. This, however, needn't be an issue. Contrary to popular belief, I am *not* a hardliner when it comes to "grafting" and putting in the hours in the gym. I believe you should be training all the time, yes, but that doesn't mean you should be going *all out* all the time. You should move every day. And frequently. But this increased frequency must be matched by a decreased intensity.

Again, we've covered this. You get it.

It's those *others*...

For the most part, I recommend taking your *existing* workout and breaking it into smaller parts. This way, you are not training more or less than you otherwise would be. You're simply spacing it out more. *Maybe* adding some additional, light volume.

I recommend that you learn your body's cues well enough to identify when you have offered sufficient stimulus for growth in some area and then take that as your cue to pause. Of course, this will change as you become more experienced.

That might mean "getting a pump," for example, or it might mean beginning to hit a wall in terms of your strength or skill. Rather than switching to the next body part or exercise at this point, you simply take your break and come back to it fresh.

But the other point is that not all exercise needs to be strength training. There is *so* much else to train, and this is the perfect opportunity to do it. For example, you can maybe fit in that mobility training you've been meaning to do. Or perhaps some skills training.

In my previous book, *Functional Training and Beyond*, I discussed the huge benefit of training with a wide range of different modalities.

Lately, I've been praising the benefits of martial arts training for non-martial artists. Throwing head-high kicks has huge value for anyone; it builds balance, mobility, strength, coordination, and more. Nearly all the best movers I've ever met have been martial artists.

You don't need to be a martial artist to practice roundhouse and spin hook kicks. It's also something you can do anywhere and it's *extremely* fun. And by breaking your workouts into smaller chunks, you'll have a much better opportunity to do this. No longer is your training.

Which brings me to the next chapter, quite nicely.

Chapter 5

INCIDENTAL TRAINING (OR LEARNING THE SPLITS WHILE BRUSHING YOUR TEETH)

Beyond merely breaking your workouts into multiple smaller sessions, you can train throughout your day by turning everyday activities into challenges. This is what I call "incidental training."

A good example might be to practice horse stance (mabu) while brushing your teeth.

Horse stance is a position from martial arts that involves widening the feet and then sitting down into that position—like a wide squat. This is a fantastic tool for stretching and opening the hips. Seeing as a lot of people have trouble with their hips, this can translate to reduced pain, higher kicks, a deeper squat, and more. Some people even progressively widen the horse stance to reach the middle splits.

Practicing horse stance strengthens tendons deep in the hips *and* trains the core. It should be practiced with the back straight, too.

For most people holding horse stance for thirty seconds can be challenging. What better opportunity than while brushing your teeth? This will allow you to build up to a full two to three minutes (the optimal toothbrushing length seems to vary from country to country).

Eventually, you could do your whole morning routine in horse stance!

Or how about using this opportunity to practice calf raises? Many people struggle with small calves, but one solution is performing a hundred calf raises every day. This is boring and difficult to remember, which is where brushing your teeth provides the perfect opportunity.

And if you find yourself forgetting? Put up a Post-it note to remind yourself.

Many more opportunities for incidental training, exercises, and drills lend themselves to this approach.

How about sitting in a gentle stretch while watching TV? You can perform calf raises on pavement while waiting for a bus. You can train your grip strength with a tennis ball while you wait for the kettle to boil. You can practice juggling while your computer loads.

Try performing slow kicks while balancing on one leg as you talk on the phone.

The Right Choices

Of course, incidental training can also mean choosing to walk instead of getting the bus (or, better yet, choosing to jog). It can mean taking the stairs instead of the elevator.

Or it can mean rethinking what to do with an evening.

For example, instead of watching television every evening, you could think of activities to get you up and moving.

A great choice for me lately has been VR. In particular, *Beat Saber*[32] gets me up and moving, burns calories, and is still fun and even addictive.

The potential of VR for training is *massive*. And we'll be coming back to this in a big way toward the end of this book.

Of course, no one became a top-performing athlete by playing *Beat Saber*. But if the options are to play *Beat Saber* or sit on the couch, the former will certainly benefit your overall health. And there are a *lot* of anecdotal cases of people losing weight and getting into great shape by simply getting good at this one game.

If nothing else, ten minutes of *Beat Saber* will help you to burn off that extra chocolate bar you shouldn't have had, given sufficient intensity.

And there are many other options, too. How about some motion-controlled games? Or even a spot of badminton in the garden with the other half? Or just a walk.

I'm not talking about exercise specifically here. I'm talking about making your leisure time more active.

You're Not Tired, You're Lethargic!

I am already anticipating the pushback on this. You're too tired to be that active in the evenings, right?

Well, my hunch is that you may not be tired so much as *lethargic*.

---

32 For those unfamiliar with it, *Beat Saber* is a virtual reality game that challenges you to hit incoming orbs in time with a music track. It's a lot of fun and can get challenging. *Pistol Whip* is also another good one!

What do I mean by this? Well, if you've been largely stationary for an entire day, it's unlikely that you're physically tired. Your glycogen stores should still be there. You probably aren't accruing microtears.

You likely aren't physically fatigued.

Even sleep deprivation has little effect on physical strength.[33]

Instead, you are likely mentally tired *or* suffering from sluggishness due to a lack of movement.

This is why if I were to ask you to do twenty push-ups *right now*, you would probably feel an intense mental block preventing you from doing that.

If you've been sitting on your behind all day in an office, chances are that you haven't engaged your glutes or quads for a while. This may lead to a loss of sensation and control in those muscles. They have effectively "gone to sleep." You feel sluggish and tired.

Your heart rate has also been slow, and circulation is likely limited.

And all this inactivity may be reflected in the brain by an overabundance of "inhibitory" neurotransmitters (rather than excitatory). The result is that engaging the glutes and driving power through the legs now appears to take much more effort than it should.

In fact, *any* kind of exercise will have that effect.

But if you get up and move, you may find that this changes. As the blood starts circulating, as you get more oxygen and blood to your muscles and

---

33   Olivia E. Knowles et al., "Inadequate sleep and muscle strength: Implications for resistance training," *J Sci Med Sport.* 21, no. 9 (2018): 959–968.

brain and regain conscious control over your muscles, you suddenly have greater energy.

It should be a warning sign that it takes us so long to warm up before a workout. Why do we need to spend hours "revving up" like a cold engine before we can use our bodies to their full extent?

According to the school of somatics, this could eventually lead to the chronic loss of control over certain muscles. This is referred to as "sensory motor amnesia." While there is still limited evidence supporting somatics, this does make a lot of intuitive sense. A lot of our awkward movement patterns occur because we use certain postures so much and others so *little*.

(It also calls to mind how I come crashing out of bed first thing in the morning, falling face-first into the wardrobe as I run to get my screaming child.)

Have you ever noticed how animals don't need to do a warm-up before they run? This is because they typically spend more time moving their bodies, so they aren't as stiff and cold before they need to move.

Instead, they perform a simple stretch—called a "pandiculation"—which is thought to help awaken those muscles via contraction and stretching.[34] Yawning is, in fact, a particular form of pandiculation believed to affect the muscles of the respiratory system, specifically. These pandiculations may also help to "restore and reset" the "structural, functional equilibrium of the myofascial system."

The point is: if you start moving, you will feel more awake. You'll increase circulation to the muscles and the brain, you'll wake up those muscles

---

34 Luiz Fernando Bertolucci, "Pandiculation: nature's way of maintaining the functional integrity of the myofascial system?," *J Bodyw Mov Ther* 15, no. 3 (2011): 268–80.

that have gone to sleep, and you'll increase excitatory neurotransmitters to put yourself in a more alert state.

The hardest part is to break the cycle when you're already tired and lethargic. And the best way to do that is to start with some light movements that you truly enjoy. That could mean a little bit of skipping, juggling, or balance board training.

Well, that's what I enjoy. Maybe you prefer doing keepy-ups. Or dancing. Or *Wii Sports*. There's *Nintendo Switch Sports*,[35] but it's not the same.

Don't try and trick yourself into doing a bigger workout. You can't trick yourself just like you can't tickle yourself. Be genuinely okay with a small activity, like a game of *Beat Saber*.

All this is *also* why exercise and movement can be powerful methods for overcoming low moods. If you're feeling low or tired, for whatever reason, the natural inclination is to "lean into it." We put on sad or slow music, sit on the sofa, and do nothing.

Instead, try revving yourself up to tackle that low mood with brute force. Dance to music. Do some shadowboxing.[36] Go for a jog. You'll feel a lot better than if you had simply given up for the day.

Better yet, if you consistently move throughout the day, you may find you don't feel so sluggish in the first place.[37]

---

35 "How to date your book before it's even published in one easy step!"

36 I've also found that when I'm anxious about an interview, test, or awkward social situation, instead of trying to "calm down" and control my breathing, I opt to *psych myself up*. There's a big, positive difference between being "psyched up" and "psyched out." For one interview, I leaned into the physiological arousal by listening to "You've Got the Touch" by Stan Bush and doing a workout. I felt ready to take on the world! (I did not get the job.)

37 This is also a good moment to share a tip from my friend, Becka. She told me that if she has anything she needs to do in an evening, she will make sure she does it *before* she eats and *before* she sits down. This makes sense, seeing as sitting down switches off the body in so many ways.

And incidental training is a great way to do that.

Adaptation Facilitation Machine

Let's engage in a thought experiment.

If I'm making the argument that you should be moving and challenging yourself throughout the day, then surely the logical extreme would be to design the environment in such a way as to be trained by sheer osmosis. Such that simply moving around your home or work environment would entail a kind of training.

This would be the closest thing to emulating the way our bodies adapted in the wild. During our evolution, simply moving barefoot on uneven terrain would have been enough to train the feet and ankles. Climbing trees and crags would build the arms and grip strength. Running after prey and walking long distances would train our endurance.

At some point, as I've discussed previously, humans gained the ability to shape and design the environment around them. The result of this? We created spaces that *coddled* us. Spaces built almost entirely for comfort removed any challenge element from our routine.

And spaces that were flat, predictable, and dull.

Is it any wonder we've lost the ability to move?

We are just as domesticated as our pet poodles. Nothing against poodles; I had two poodles and I loved them to bits.

But...y'know.

We could even argue that maintaining a consistent temperature could be bad for our bodies. The same with consistent lighting. Some research is now suggesting that keeping the windows open and maintaining a less sterile environment could prevent disease by allowing a better balance of good and bad bacteria.

Those topics are a little beyond the scope of this book for now, however.

I'm not suggesting we all start living outside again. That comes with disadvantages.

Instead, seeing as we can now design our environments, we could start thinking about how to make them *even better* at making us stronger *without* many downsides.

Can we do one better than nature?

In my last book, I called such a location the "Adaptation Facilitation Machine," inspired by Cal Newport's "Eudaimonia Machine."

For example, we might start with the front door, a heavy door that can be pushed or pulled open. You must then jump a small height over the step and inside. The hall branches off in two directions. One room has a low door that requires you to stoop or crawl to get in. The other has a high door that you must step/vault over.

The living room has monkey bars on the ceiling.[38] You can use these to get to wherever you need. There's also a balance beam running along the middle of the room. Instead of sofas, you're encouraged to sit on the floor or squat. The floor itself is uneven.

---

38 I did warn you...

To get upstairs, you need to do some bouldering. There is a bucket and pulley in case you need to carry anything. A second option would be to climb a rope.

You get the idea.

Now, of course, this isn't a particularly practical solution in real life. A few people have already pointed out to me that such a house would be dangerous in case of a fire. Guests wouldn't be particularly eager to come and visit,[39] and you would struggle if you were ever to get injured.

If we wanted to make something like this work, we'd need to take these practical considerations into account. There would need to be an alternate option for getting about, for getting furniture upstairs. But we would need to ensure that there was proper incentive to not *always* use this easier option. Perhaps it would lack the perks of the rest of the home. There would need to be emergency exits and perhaps scaffolding for furnishing the upstairs.

Of course, this is not how I live. While I might like to, I'm not sure my wife would be on-board with the idea. It's generally impractical.

But I think these ideas will *one day* factor into how we think about our homes. Instead of asking, "How can we make this home as comfortable as possible?" we should instead ask what adaptations a space will bring about in a person.

A couple of realistic changes we could make to our environments right now would be to:

- Remove a lot of the comfortable furniture (something a friend of mine has done)

---

39   Perhaps this is a positive?

- Avoid placing items on cupboards and place them either low down or high up to encourage more movement. Low cupboards are the way forward.

- Employ less even terrain—in the garden, at least

- Make doors a little heavier and stiffer

- Make each step a little taller

Opportunities to Move

Another option is to create "opportunities to move" around the house and office.

My office has dip bars, a balance board, juggling balls, a skipping rope, and dumbbells. Likewise, my house has a pull-up bar, a rope for climbing, and parallettes. The living room has a balance beam that can be folded away when not in use. At one point, I kept a kettlebell by the stairs and made the rule that I had to carry it up and down the stairs every time I made the trip either way.

These opportunities are optional, but they provide a sufficient stimulus, nonetheless.

Often, I'll feel stiff in the office, get up and play on the balance board, then sit back down to carry on typing.

Why not keep a balance board by the sink in the kitchen?

It will also create a unique appearance for your décor.

One of the most important changes you can make to your home, though? Create some wide-open space.

Unfortunately, modern interior design does not think this way. In fact, the object is to use all the space in a "practical" way. Unused space is referred to as "unresolved."

Worse, open space is even missing from *gyms* a lot of the time, making the mistake of cramming in as much equipment as humanly possible.

Open space is necessary for *truly* using your body. Whether it's for running, cartwheels, practicing tornado kicks, walking on your hands, crawling, or doing animal flow. Having a bare wall is a great idea, too, for kicking up to a handstand or stretching your arms.

To me this should be obvious: if you want to train and use your body to its fullest, you *need space*.

Changing Your Relationship with the Environment

More than changing the space around you, it's about changing your *relationship* with that space.

You don't *need* a climbing wall on your stairs. You can just as easily challenge yourself to jump up the stairs three at a time. Or to jump *down* the stairs.

Notice how we're essentially learning to move like children again. This is something innate we all start with but unfortunately "unlearn" as we get older…and more boring.

You can make a rule to perform a calf raise on each step.

You can challenge yourself to turn the light switches on and off with your feet: something that requires balance, control, and mobility. Try and open the pot of tuna paste with one hand.

(I love tuna paste.)

"Environment" doesn't just mean the space around you in this context; it also means your habits within that space.

The real secret to an effective adaptation facilitation machine is a bit of imagination and *lots* of Post-it notes.

Because perhaps surprisingly, one of the hardest parts about doing this is *remembering* to do it.

Chapter 6

THE FUNDAMENTAL HUMAN MOVEMENTS

Okay, let's return to Earth for a moment.

You do not live in a future home designed to try and kill you. (A good thing.)

And most people do not train using sufficient variety or frequency to optimize performance. (A genuinely bad thing.)

Right now, our environments shape us in an entirely passive manner.

So, what are the results? What specifically is this damaging?

Overall, the issue here is what's *missing*. In a more natural environment, we would have used a far greater range of movements than we do now. And each movement would have had far more variety and far more nuance.

Variety is key here. Because sitting in and of itself is not awful. It's not an ideal posture, but it wouldn't kill you if you did it for an hour or so a day.

The problem is that we often do so little else.

The natural environment is important to consider, as it is the environment we evolved to suit. It is the environment *that evolved us*.

But that doesn't mean we need to fully embrace the meme and "return to monkey."

There is no "perfect environment" for the human animal. After all, the only constant in the environment is how much it has changed. Humans have travelled, the climate has changed, and different cultures lived entirely differently.

Evolution is in a state of permaflux. We might seem "out of time," but we always were.

There are only a few exceptions here, those being animals that have almost perfectly adapted to a generally static environment. Like sharks, apparently.

Bloody sharks.

We could, however, argue that our environment has changed *particularly* quickly in recent years. This is why we still seem unsuited for our modern lifestyles.

And again, it has changed *unnaturally*. We have forged the environment with no mind to how that might impact our health.

So, what fundamental movements has the human body evolved to perform? What's missing from the average movement diet?

And what can we do about it?

Codifying Human Movement

There have been many attempts to codify optimal human movement in this way. The fact that they're all so different should tell us something about how successful they have been.

But there are several common suggestions and logical assumptions.

One of the most often cited lists of "necessary" movements for the prototypical human comes from Paul Chek. Paul describes the following seven primal movements:

- Squat
- Pull
- Gait (walking, jogging, running)
- Lunge
- Bend
- Push
- Twist

Paul did not simply pull these ideas out of thin air but came to his conclusions after studying the development of infants. Which movements do they learn first and why? Which ones seem to be almost hardwired?

The only issue with this list is it provides broad categories. "Gait" could mean running, walking, or jogging. All of these are slightly different. Bending could mean bending the spine or hinging at the hips. Twisting could mean twisting the upper body or the hips (something that martial artists consider in detail).

It also misses combinations of movements. For example, throwing is a kind of back extension and twist. Jumping is a squat and a hip hinge with added dorsiflexion.

These are certainly "fundamental," however.

One way we could break these down further could be to consider the basic *activities* that are universally required among humans. By moving up a level to the broader movement goals, we can better grasp what we are specifically required to do.

This list, unsurprisingly, is a lot longer.

- Walk
- Jog
- Sprint
- Jump
- Bend
- Pull
- Push
- Handle
- Rend (pull apart, push together)
- Raise (i.e., raise an object to your face)
- Squat
- Carry
- Sit
- Lay down
- Scramble
- Roll

- Get up
- Throw
- Direction change
- Climb/Hang/Brachiate
- Slope ascend
- Slope descend
- Kneel
- Crawl
- Lunge
- Balance
- Swim

I argue that these are "fundamental human movements." We need to do all these things to be considered functional individuals, which are broadly universal. Everyone will at some point need to manipulate an object, throw something, or climb.

Breaking down movement this way is at once more generic *and* more specific.

But it's by no means comprehensive. It is, in fact, still arbitrary.

And that's the nature of the beast, I think. That's what I've been saying: our natural movement is far *too* broad and varied. We are too adaptable.

We are *beyond* categorization.

Still, these are the movements that likely would have been required of us during our evolution. Therefore, our bodies evolved, *assuming* that we were performing them.

When we *stop* performing any of these things, we create an imbalance. Muscles that developed for specific functions now have little purpose.

Thus, they atrophy—and their contributions to our overall structural integrity (and tensegrity) are minimized. Meanwhile, other activities we overuse end up pulling us in different directions and create focussed areas of tension.

An example of something many of us are missing is swimming. Ben Patrick recommends performing the tibialis raise to strengthen the tibialis anterior. This is a muscle of the shin that is responsible for dorsiflexion. According to Ben, training this muscle will help to absorb the impact from running and jumping, preventing shin splints and avoiding injury.

But the tibialis raise, which involves resting on the heels and raising the toes, looks like the most *unnatural* movement you could perform. Why do we need this if, presumably, it's something we would never have trained naturally?

Prehistoric man did *not* do tibialis raises. No, I don't have evidence for this. I'm just not having it. Nope.

So, how can we say we need it? Did prehistoric man struggle with shin splints?

Well, one way we would have trained it is by swimming. When we swim, we need to dorsiflex or create an isometric contraction in the anterior tibialis to propel ourselves through the water.

There are other ways we can get this naturally, as I already listed. Things like hill sprints (or jogging uphill). Trail running, more generally.

Likewise, it always seemed odd that it's so *easy* to create a shoulder impingement by pressing overhead with a slight interior rotation. Why would the body be arranged so we can easily injure ourselves with a seemingly basic movement?

Well, it turns out that the shoulders might be naturally remedied through climbing and hanging. Hanging from a bar overhead might help physically move the acromion and reshape the coracoacromial ligament, opening the space and minimizing the risk of impingement. This is according to author Dr. John Kirsch.

Conversely, sitting and hunching forward for hours on end every day might be what closed it up in the first place.

The body, as a system, is built on the assumption that you will sometimes climb and/or hang. As we saw earlier, this is not a modern pastime. It is something we have done for centuries.

Jumping and running regularly will increase bone density. Natural movement provides the right balance of different activities to create a well-rounded physique and minimize pain and loss of movement.

In short: movement is medicine. As long as it's the right movement in the right quantities provided by simply existing in a dynamic environment.

The Problem with Training "Everything"

While I'd love to tell you I've achieved the impossible and found the universal theory of human movement, the truth is that this is still an arbitrary list. Throwing means what? Shotput throw? Underarm throw? Underarm throw?

Carrying means what? Carrying a bowl of water on your head? Carrying a child on your front?

Jumping means what? Jumping from one leg or two?

And, as we've discussed, *every* jump is different, especially on natural terrain.

And what of those unexpected situations? Like when you find yourself jumping up to your wardrobe and darting your hand forward at the apex of that jump to grab something? You know what I mean.

The truth is I don't believe in neatly codifying human movement. I don't believe in Occam's Razor.

I'm not a minimalist. I'm a maximalist.

There *is* no convenient list of all movement, which I'll get to in more detail in a moment.

What We Don't Need

I think what's interesting to consider is what we *don't* need. Where does our training miss the mark?

In my opinion, *far* too much emphasis is placed on strength training regarding performance and health.

To be clear, I have nothing but respect for people who can bench press, squat, or deadlift huge numbers. I have a good bench press that I'm proud of (about 150 kilograms 1RM on a good day).

And I enjoy doing it.

But this is a sport and a sport only. It does not translate, beyond a certain point, to overall performance.

For starters, movements like the bench press and the squat will never be directly useful. I can bench press 150 kilograms, sure. But what if I tried to push 150 kilograms? Chances are my body weight would move backward. I'm too light to push this much.

Therefore, I would never need to be that strong in the chest and shoulders. Instead, it would make more sense to use a cable press from a standing position and to thereby use the entire body as one functional unit, something J.C. Santana, from the Institute of Human Performance, put me onto.

Matters are made worse by the fact that powerlifters are taught to retract the shoulder blades while pressing—something that you would never naturally do—and to arch their backs to limit the range of motion. This is a sport, not a guide to optimal performance.

The same goes for squats. Squatting places a huge compressive load on the spine, and for what? You would never be able to lift something that heavy onto your back, so why would you need to squat with it?

This is not to say squatting isn't valuable—it's amazing for improving jump height and much more. But if you can already squat double body weight, you will experience diminishing returns by simply trying to lift *even more*.

Even the deadlift, arguably one of the most functional movements in the world, has its limitations. Deadlifts teach us to pick a straight bar up off the flat ground. That bar is raised to a convenient level and the movement is near-identical every time.

This is different from picking up a sock, a log, a human being, a piece of furniture, or anything else. Even a tyre flip shows how different "real" lifting is: as you need to widen your stance to get close enough to the tyre, deal with an entirely different "strength curve,"[40] and hinge/squat much lower down to get your fingers under the tyre.

There will likely be some rounding of the back during this process—which is something a lot of powerlifters get distressed by. But again, this is life. When lifting a pram out of a car boot or placing a child into a cot, you *will* need to round your back. When lifting a sofa from the ground, you *will* need to round your back.

When people assert that "hinging is the correct way to pick something up from the floor," I'm always confused. Says who? When have you ever seen *anyone* naturally deadlift an item off the floor? Are we to believe that our bodies move incorrectly when we let them do their own thing? This is true even as a child—it's not the result of conditioning by our modern lifestyles.

The key is not to hide from this type of movement but rather to integrate it gently and use higher rep ranges and lighter loads to strengthen the connective tissue in these more vulnerable positions to make them *invulnerable*.

---

40 The weight of the tyre changes as you balance it upright.

The Problem with Perfect Form

This is the problem with trying to codify human movement or trying to achieve the perfect form on any given lift.

There is no perfect form because the environment changes. The perfect form should arrange itself around the demands of the environment and the goal.

Being highly adaptable is the end goal of a true all-around athlete. And it's the only way to fortify against serious injury.

We need to prepare the body for those inconvenient positions that we can hardly anticipate with light, controlled loads: ready for when the situations inevitably arise out of our control.

We therefore need what Nicolai Bernstein refers to as "repetition without repetition."

And this benefits performance, too. Remember our study from earlier?

(Cue harp music.)

"More variability in practice conditions" could help baseball batters to better solve coordination challenges and thus, improve performance.

Black Box Training

Ultimately, I am recommending we embrace our ignorance. We bow to the sheer complexity and ingenuity of the human body and stop trying to "hack" it into greater performance. We respect the human body for what it is: a black box.

There is simply too much going on here. There are too many adaptations. Heck, we only discovered the role of the fascia recently! What else is going on under the hood?

Rather than trying to second-guess the "optimal" movement and neatly codify it, we should feed the body the input it needs and let it do the rest.

One way we can do this is by turning activity into exercise.

Here's the perfect example: rock climbing.

Rock Climbing Is the Ultimate Pull Workout

Earlier, I discussed how climbing a tree was a more comprehensive pull workout versus doing pull-ups. This is true because every branch is different and reaching for different branches will subtly alter the effort you need to exert.

This doesn't quite work. Most trees aren't built like ladders. You'll be supporting your weight on your legs a lot of the time. And you won't have far to climb, in most cases.

Bouldering is different. Bouldering is a form of rock climbing that sees you climbing short distances without a rope over a crash mat (usually). This can be performed at a climbing centre or on real-world "crags."

This creates a better opportunity to perform a range of pulling movements.

Simply bouldering a lot can build some of the most performant upper body pulling strength possible.

My suggestion is to approach this slightly differently, though. Instead of rock climbing with the intent of *getting to the top of the crag*, you could instead rock climb with the intent of training the upper body.

In other words: increase resistance by relying entirely, or mostly, on the arms. Reach for holds that challenge you (rather than taking the most strategic route to the top from the perspective of someone trying to climb *well*).

Repeat movements. Go up and down multiple times and try to "feel the burn" in the muscles working.

In short, you are climbing with the goal of fitness rather than climbing to the top. And this is a perfect example of what I described earlier as **Black Box Training** because you are simply providing the body with a dynamic and chaotic form of resistance without worrying about technique on a repetitive lift.

More Examples

There are *many* more examples of this. For example, wrestling is often praised for its strength-building benefits. This builds strength, endurance, rotational power, explosive strength, core strength, and more.

Again, wrestling is something we might well have done in various forms during our natural evolution. Funny that!

Again, you can wrestle in a manner that isn't about defeating the opponent but rather *both* getting good training. Spending half an hour wrestling would be an incredible way to develop extremely transferable strength, endurance, and mental fortitude. And, like climbing, it would be more fun than lifting weights.

Speaking of martial arts, bag work and kicking are also perfect. Or sparring. Or how about dance? Where, again, the aim is to perform the moves that most severely challenge your balance, strength, and endurance?

Dance is universal across cultures and dates back seemingly to the origins of humanity.

Or how about trail running? Running on uneven terrain will develop stability and strength in the lower legs, alongside balance, in a manner you can't accomplish from squats and other movements.

We've seen that swimming can strengthen the tibialis anterior, but that's just scratching the surface of what this amazing exercise can do.

Slacklining has been shown to provide countless benefits in terms of running speed, jumping height, and ground-contact time.[41] Just *balancing on stuff* is exceptionally good for us. And you can check my last book for a deeper dive into that.

This is the art of using activities and hobbies as your main form of fitness. But this doesn't apply to all forms of exercise. While riding a bike or rowing a boat are no doubt good for you, they also involve repetitive movements in a linear pattern.

Specifically, what I'm focussing on here are movements that involve larger degrees of freedom. Activities repetitive enough to offer some stimulus while offering a far more comprehensive strengthening of not just the target muscles but the entire surrounding connective tissue.

---

41   Javier Fernández-Rio et al., "Effects of Slackline Training on Acceleration, Agility, Jump Performance and Postural Control in Youth Soccer Players," *J Hum Kinet* 67 (2019): 235–245; Jürgen Pfusterschmied et al., "Effects of 4-week slackline training on lower limb joint motion and muscle activation," *J Sci Med Sport* 16, no. 6 (2013): 562–6.

Chapter 7

KEEPING YOUR BRAIN ACTIVE

In the last chapter, I described some of what's "missing" from regular training programs and modern lifestyles. I also discussed some of the things we need to seek: the "fundamental human movements" and properties we have lost in many cases.

We also saw that some of the aspects of fitness that we covet aren't all that important in the grand scheme of things.

But one aspect of our performance has taken perhaps the biggest hit of all: the cognitive aspect.

That is to say that our training should also involve our *brains*. And our lifestyles should involve varied challenges for our brains, too.

In the opening chapter of this book, I celebrated the apparent wonder of the human body. But before you get too pleased with yourself, consider that we are in many ways *drastically inferior* to many of our animal relatives.

We think we are the most intelligent and advanced species on the planet, mainly because we are biased to value precisely the traits we possess.

But what if I told you that chimpanzees have far superior working memories? When given tasks that involve memorizing the positions of shapes on a screen, chimpanzees can respond *significantly faster* and *significantly* more accurately than humans.[42]

One common explanation is that humans have gone through a kind of "trade-off." The idea is that we have swapped a near-photographic memory for our more useful abstract reasoning.

I'm not convinced. Who says that cognitive functions are an either/or thing? Why did we swap that ability specifically?

Rather, what if the reason we stopped being able to identify patterns of objects at a glance is because we stopped *training* this ability?

Think about the life of a chimpanzee: constantly swinging through trees, balancing along branches, keeping track of prey, considering the positions of the other chimps...

Tracking objects and predicting their movements is their bread and butter.

We've seen how the Aboriginal members of NORFORCE in the Australian outback can see better than average humans, and we can assume this is due to their natural requirement to stay vigilant.

Many indigenous tribes are incredible trackers, and stories abound of how they can even outperform modern technology when wayfinding.

---

42   Tetsuro Matsuzawa, "Cognitive development in chimpanzees: A trade-off between memory and abstraction?," in *The Making of Human Concepts*, ed. Denis Mareschal, Paul C. Quinn, & Stephen E. G. Lea, 227–244. Oxford University Press.

So, is it that far-fetched to think that a similar lifestyle might favour an effective visual working memory? And could some of this be relearned?

While there's not much research on the matter, there is little to suggest that indigenous tribes at least have a slightly different approach to tasks involving working memory.[43]

The notion that lifestyle and adaptive training give chimpanzees their remarkable abilities—at least to some extent—makes even more sense when considering how working memory works.

Working Memory: It's Kind of a Big Deal

Working memory is the memory store we use when holding onto information to manipulate it or use it later. The example often given is remembering a phone number while looking for a pen to write it down. We also use this when carrying over numbers during mental arithmetic.

Traditionally, working memory was described as having a capacity of seven, plus or minus two. This is to say that someone with a good working memory could recall nine numbers, while someone with a poor working memory could only manage five.

The truth, of course, is *far* more complex.

---

43   Melissa R. Freire & Kristen Pammer, "Influence of culture on visual working memory: evidence of a cultural response bias for remote Australian Indigenous children," *Journal of Cultural Cognitive Science* 4, no. 4 (2020): 323–341.

Because we use our working memories all the time and across multiple modalities. For example, you use working memory when playing sports[44] and trying to remember the positions of all the other players on the pitch.

And you use working memory during conversation to think of what you will say next while remembering the context and what has already been said.

Moreover, you use working memory to construct your visuospatial experience of the world. Everything you perceive exists in working memory.

Far too much information enters our brain through our senses for us to possibly make use of it. Thus, we only truly attend to a small piece of that information at any given time: we focus on a small detailed "keyhole image" of the world at the centre of our focus (at the fovea, which has a much sharper resolution than our peripheral vision).

The brain then pieces these glimpses together to create the *impression* of a wider and more broadly detailed scene. Gaps in our awareness (due to "inattentional blindness") are filled in with assumptions, schemas, and longer-term memories. You don't see the whole canvas; you imagine that you do.

You are not experiencing the world as it is, then, but as a facsimile constructed from snapshots and held together in working memory. Thus, our working memory and our visuospatial landscape are closely related.

This process results in some real deficits and flaws in perception. For one, our perception does not include accurate, up-to-date information that we

44   Laure Pisella, "Visual perception is dependent on visuospatial working memory and thus on the posterior parietal cortex," Annals of Physical and Rehabilitation Medicine 60, no. 3 (2017):141–147.

haven't been focussed on. Gaps in attention can lead to issues if we're in a sports competition or driving.

A famous psychological demonstration tasks viewers to follow a team of individuals playing catch with a ball and to catch how many times the ball is successfully passed. When questioned, most participants fail to notice the gorilla that walks casually into the shot, waves, then walks off-screen.

Vision tests may not be enough to truly sess the usefulness of the visual system as they leave this important element out. And as we age, our visual perception and processing power decrease.

Fortunately, plasticity can occur within the visual cortex, and it is possible to *improve* both perception in the peripheral vision *and* visual processing.[45]

Thus, 3D object-tracking tools and other methods exist for training these abilities: things that are already *naturally* trained by the natural environment and the increased perception and awareness that novel locations promote.

These tools are often employed in virtual reality and task users with tracking and reacting to different moving objects in their visual field. They are somewhat useful for helping to improve sports performance[46]— though more research is still needed.

I created a working memory tool called "BioMind," which you can download from my website for free.

---

45 Jyoti Mishra et al., "Neural Plasticity Underlying Visual Perceptual Learning in Aging," *Brain Res* 1612 (2016):140–151; Elisa Castaldi, "Neuroplasticity in adult human visual cortex," *Neuroscience & Biobehavioral Reviews* 112 (2020): 542–552.

46 Thomas Romeas et al., "3D-Multiple Object Tracking training task improves passing decision-making accuracy in soccer players," *Psychology of Sport and Exercise* 22 (2015):1–9.

Or we can try and train the working memory directly. And theoretically, this could improve many aspects of our performance by allowing us to process more information of every kind.

How Working Memory Works and How to Improve It

To improve working memory, we should first consider how it works.

Unfortunately, as is often the case, we're not sure.

It is generally agreed that there is no single "store" for working memory corresponding to a particular brain region. This once seemed to be the case, based on descriptions of working memory such as the "visuospatial scratchpad."

Instead, we now think that working memory results from persistent activity across neurons without external stimuli. That is to say that when we hold onto the image of a loved one, we do so by activating similar brain networks to those that would be active when seeing them. This continuous activity may be maintained via "re-entrant loops." That is to say that the brain maintains activity by creating a kind of circuit. We may experience this consciously when we rehearse a phone number by repeating it to ourselves.

This further suggests that working memory is dispersed across multiple different brain regions. And while some brain areas are commonly implicated in working memory (frontal and posterior brain areas with support from subcortical structures),[47] it's highly likely that the *precise* brain areas are dictated by the nature of the task at home.

This is referred to as the component process's view of working memory. And this description makes sense considering everything we have discussed so far. And it is backed by case studies of individuals experiencing damage to specific brain regions, resulting in impaired brain function in specific types of working memory. It also explains why athletes, for example, are more likely to use their kinaesthetic rather than visual senses when mentally rotating 3D objects, as we previously saw.

There are competing theories of working memory. Some are "activity silent" (meaning that the neurons are not required to keep firing) and rely on fast Hebbian plasticity on a timescale of milliseconds. That is to say that the brain could be rewiring itself in real time as you think. Perhaps short-term plasticity could also play a role as certain networks become more likely to fire following activity.

Whatever the case, however, it seems that working memory takes place across the brain. We must therefore train multiple brain regions and the connectivity between those brain regions.

Tools like dual N-Back can be useful but are limited in scope because they train specific working memory in specific brain regions. 3D object trackers are better, but they're still limited compared to how we use our brains every day.

Instead, we should look for methods that combine different types of working memory across different modalities, working in different ways. And these methods should challenge not only the ability to store lots

47   Johan Eriksson et al., "Neurocognitive architecture of working memory," *Neuron* 88, no. 1 (2016): 33–46.

of information but also the ability to quickly switch between tasks and maintain storage in the face of distraction.

And the best way to achieve this? Engage in dynamic tasks in a shifting and changing environment.

The parallels with "functional training" are quite fascinating. For example, many training methods focusing on strength or muscle building use linear movements that don't engage other systems. These can improve performance but only to a certain extent.

Dual N-Back is effective, just like a bicep curl is effective. But the more "compound" and truly functional exercise might be more dynamic in both cases.

The best way to train for a sport or activity is to engage in that sport or activity. We adapt to the lifestyles we lead. And unfortunately, these are static with minimal dynamic movement.

Unfortunately, something similar is going on for the brain, too. We rarely are tasked with focussing on one thing for long. The internet provides us with all the information we could need at our fingertips—all in bite-sized, consumable form. Our attention is constantly pulled one way and another.

When we *do* use our brains, it is typically while seated, looking directly forward at a computer screen. Or, in the best-case scenario, a car windshield.

Rarely do we engage in cognitively demanding, novel tasks that we aren't already used to.

Now consider the lifestyle of hunter-gatherers who would constantly need to consider the locations of their fellow humans. Who would need

to be aware of their surroundings when tracking prey and looking for food. Who would discover new places and feel their brains flood with plasticity-enhancing chemicals.

Who would have no help from a calendar, calculator, diary, GPS device, or another form of "exocortex."

They would use their brains in a moving, dynamic, and three-dimensional manner.

This is where sports can provide a fantastic alternative: keeping track of moving objects in the environment while juggling different tasks and goals is like tracking food, friends, and foes.

Studies support the idea: elite athletes demonstrate improved working memory versus the general population or even amateur athletes.[48] Again, some of the best training comes from what we consider to be a "hobby" rather than a dedicated "workout."

It makes a *lot* of intuitive sense to think that team sports should be so good for us.

"Fixing" the Brain Using Adaptive Training

Short of becoming an elite athlete or, I guess, a chimpanzee, what can we do to challenge our working memories?

48   Robert S Vaughan et al., "Attention, working-memory control, working-memory capacity, and sport performance: The moderating role of athletic expertise," *Eur J Sport Sci* 21, no. 2 (2021): 240–249.

One option is to challenge the brain with moving tasks. Proprioceptive tasks that involve moving in 3D space inherently utilize far more information as the body needs to consider the position of all its limbs, how they relate to the environment around them, and how this all relates to the visual information coming in.

This is why studies suggest that proprioceptive tasks like climbing trees, balancing on beams, and more can have a dramatic, beneficial impact on measures of cognitive performance, such as working memory.[49] It's also why something like juggling, which has been shown in many studies to boost working memory-related traits,[50] can be so effective.

You can take this further by learning to juggle on a balance board.

But will this positively impact our ability to remember names? To *do* the chores we said we'd do? To drive confidently while making the best decisions on the road?

To handle *any* large cognitive load, even when tired or stressed?

My recommendation is to train with multiple different types of brain training. Just as you don't perform a single exercise and expect this to boost your performance across the entire spectrum of physical ability.

How about dual N-Back (or BioMind) *and* juggling on a balance board? How about juggling on a balance board while performing mental arithmetic?

---

49 Ross G. Alloway and Tracy Packiam Alloway, "The Working Memory Benefits of Proprioceptively Demanding Training: A Pilot Study," *Perceptual and Motor Skills* 120, no. 3 (2015).

50 Bogdan Draganski et al., "Changes in grey matter induced by training," *Neuroplasticity* 427 (2004): 311–312.

My last book discussed the importance of training with "directive" meditation and more open "non-directive" forms.

I also recommend injecting more of these kinds of challenges into your daily life. Incidental training can apply to the brain as well as the body. So, why not keep a set of juggling balls on your desk? Or a Rubik's cube?

Keep learning.

Staying Engaged

One of the biggest challenges to training, for many people, is that it is "boring."

I would suggest that this boredom is responsible for a *lot* of problems affecting a lot of people.

Exercise, though, should not be the problem. It should be the solution.

And if you're finding your training boring, you are not getting as much out of it as you could be. This is not a platitude: it's science. When you are engaged and focused, this makes you more plastic. You learn more and faster.

The fact that training is often perceived as boring is a big red flag. What animal willingly devotes time to something they find boring that doesn't immediately offer tangible benefits?

Our emotions exist to guide us toward beneficial activities. Curling for ten minutes is not all that beneficial to the human animal.

Of course, I believe in the merit of working toward a goal. And sometimes that means doing things you'd rather not.

But I think training should be fun and should be engaging. And that means it should involve a *cognitive* element as well. It should be mentally stimulating and involve *some* kind of learning. This is what puts the brain in a more plastic state. This is what helps us learn better via the interference principle. This is what boosts the working memory. This is what makes us inherently enjoy the task at hand.

What is "fun" to your brain? Simple: it's learning.

We've grown up thinking of learning as the most boring thing we can do, but that's only because we're used to learning in such an abstract and stilted manner in classrooms from textbooks. Computer games, on the other hand, represent a much more potent example of learning. To make a computer game fun, the designers must create levels that offer the right amount of challenge without becoming too difficult. They must then ramp up the difficulty gradually to create the perfect "difficulty curve" that matches the player's increasing competence.[51]

In short, games need to keep the player learning, whether learning the rules and systems of the game or learning the reflexes to input the correct sequences of button presses.

This is what exercising *should* be like. This is why the natural state of training is *play*. Climbing trees, balancing on beams, playing sports, wrestling—these are all examples of training that involve elements of both learning and play.

---

51 And wouldn't you know, I wrote a book about computer game design a few years back. For anyone who
    wants to check it out, it's called: *Learn Unity for Android Game Development: A Guide to Game Design,
    Development, and Marketing.*

Some of the principles we've discussed take care of this automatically.

For example:

- By turning everyday tasks into training and training throughout the day, we make otherwise "dull" tasks a lot more interesting.

- By training with more variables in more dynamic environments, we make every workout slightly different and thus more engaging. Doing pull-ups from a tree branch is more interesting.

- By using sets of varying exercises—rather than precisely the same movement—we keep things more fresh and interesting.

- By training with activities and hobbies—such as climbing and swimming—we get fitness from something we enjoy.

This is also why I particularly enjoy training with calisthenics. At least at a certain point in your journey, calisthenics involves a *lot* of learning, as you must balance your body in a handstand or planche, listen to proprioceptive feedback, and learn new moves. Creating flows between different exercises is also a lot of fun, which is where kettlebell training or "movement training"[52] can be so effective.

Later in this book, you'll also encounter some examples of fitness games that you can play with a partner.

In the future, I think virtual reality will take care of the "gamification" of fitness. I believe this will be the "killer app" that makes virtual reality finally a staple of entertainment. And when this happens, I think the fitness of the average individual will be drastically "levelled up." More on this in Chapter 10.

But meanwhile, how can we go about "levelling up" right now?

---

52 Such as Animal Flow or the teachings of Ido Portal.

Chapter 8

UNDERSTANDING HYPERTROPHY AND THE "PERFECT DOSAGE"

This may all seem like a lot of theory. How are we going to turn these concepts into practical training advice? How do we make this into a workout?

On the face of it, you might think I'm suggesting that we do far less *actual* training. If our bodies largely reflect our routines, then moving in various ways throughout the day is enough to maintain optimal health.

Well, yes, this is true.

But if this "training" is so good for you, why aren't manual labourers built like bodybuilders?

Why aren't they winning sporting events?

And if sports off the best way to train working memory and focus, why aren't football players winning Nobel prizes?

First: I'd like to remind everyone that the goal here is *not* to become a super-athlete in any one area. Specialisation to that extent is to be admired, but it is not an example of optimal health for the average person.

But I do take this point: a lot of people want to be more than "healthy." People who truly love fitness and *performance* want to run faster, jump higher, lift more, think faster, and *look bigger*.

As do I.

As I said in my last book and repeatedly on my website: I don't just want to be healthy. I don't want to be able to do the things I need to be able to do.

I don't want to be functional.

I want to be SuperFunctional.

In that case, we need to up the intensity. And here's how we do that.

Understanding Hypertrophy

To turn all this theory into a real training program, we need to look at hypertrophy, adaptation, and how it works. How do we build muscle and how do we get stronger? What are the necessary inputs and stimuli that trigger desirable changes in the body?

Well, you're never going to believe this, *but*…we have no idea.

Contrary to many articles and videos that make hypertrophy sound like a simple process, the truth is that we simply don't *know* how the body transforms itself in response to training. Not in any kind of comprehensive manner, anyway.

But, as with understanding working memory, we can look at what we *do* know. We can examine the best theories. And we can take this knowledge and work with it.

Now, things are going to get a little bit technical here. But stick with me because all this science will help us build an actual program that puts all this theorizing into action. And understanding why things work is what allows us to be adaptable and alter the programs to better suit our needs.

Myofibrilla vs. Sarcoplasmic Hypertrophy

Many bodybuilding websites will break muscle building down into two simple processes: myofibrilla and sarcoplasmic hypertrophy. Often, you will hear that powerlifting builds myofibrilla hypertrophy and bodybuilding builds sarcoplasmic hypertrophy. The truth is that both do both, only to differing degrees.

Sarcoplasmic hypertrophy describes the breakdown of muscle caused by tiny microtears. Muscle is made up of microscopic muscle fibers (cells) that contain sarcomeres. Imagine sarcomeres like little telescopic poles made from "contractile proteins" capable of sliding over each other (actin and myosin). It is the compression of these poles that ultimately leads to the contraction of a muscle on the macroscopic scale.

Sarcomeres are arranged end-to-end (in series) and side-by-side (in parallel). Interestingly, training with more eccentric (lengthening) movements seems to increase sarcomeres in series. Conversely, training with more *concentric* movements will train sarcomeres in parallel.

This increase occurs as, after enough repetitious movement and stress, we begin to cause damage to these fibers; in the same way that continuously stretching and releasing an elastic band will cause it to become frayed, eventually. This damage triggers inflammation, bringing cytokines and inflammatory cells to the site. This is the same process that occurs during an injury.

These chemicals stimulate nearby satellite cells, which fuse to the muscle fibers, adding more myonuclei to trigger more protein synthesis. Myonuclei are the "CPUs" of the cell that contain the DNA and trigger the creation of new proteins. Each myonuclei has a set "domain" or area of effect, so the more you have, the more muscle mass you're capable of building.

The best way to trigger this kind of myofibrilla hypertrophy is by training with heavy weights, slow eccentrics, and lower rep counts.

Sarcoplasmic hypertrophy, on the other hand, happens when the muscle cells become more swollen with fluid and other important chemicals. Training with longer rep ranges and lower weights will typically trigger less muscle damage but will encourage "metabolic stress." This describes the build-up of metabolites within the muscles that can contribute to the familiar burning sensation and, ultimately, muscle failure.[53]

This seems to increase the fluid and metabolic products within the muscle cells: glycogen, water, sarcoplasmic reticulum (storage units for calcium), t-tubules, triglycerides (needed to produce ATP), and even

---

53   Though, of course, we don't know the *precise* mechanisms for muscle failure, either.

mitochondria (the energy factories for the cell). This is often described as muscle "swelling."

Some commenters would have you believe that myofibrilla hypertrophy is the more "real" form of hypertrophy. That bodybuilders who train for sarcoplasmic hypertrophy are "swelling" the muscles and thus building "fake" muscle. This is untrue. The body does not deal in pointless adaptations. It is not interested in building muscle for the sake of filling out a t-shirt. If your biceps are bigger, they must be able to do more. Especially considering the high metabolic demand of such muscle!

What *is* true is that myofibrilla hypertrophy contributes more to max strength, whereas sarcoplasmic hypertrophy is more important for strength endurance and work capacity. The latter is just as important and "functional." As I've already mentioned, we rarely ever need to be strong "just once."

And, after all, both types of hypertrophies are present in *all* training. Bodybuilders are strong. Trust me.

Mechanical Tension

Alongside metabolic stress and muscle damage, mechanical tension is often listed as the third crucial stimulus for triggering muscle growth. This simply means putting the muscle under a load. Even without muscle damage or metabolic build-up, this still triggers *some* muscle growth.

This is thought to be the result of mechanoreceptors. These sensors in the muscle contribute to our sense of proprioception by detecting the intensity of mechanical pressure (such as the Golgi tendon organ and muscle spindles—we met those guys earlier). They allow us to gauge our effort level, but they also trigger protein synthesis, even in the absence of other factors[54] (like increasing testosterone).

How precisely does all this work, you ask? This is a deep rabbit hole with a number of explanations. One candidate is the lipid bilayer, composed of lipid molecules that can become ruptured during tension. This could result in a cascade of chemical processes, leading ultimately to increased protein synthesis. Interestingly, different kinds of mechanoreceptors may react to different types of stress on the muscle.

Blood Supply and Satellite Cell Count

These three forms of hypertrophy are the ones that get by *far* the most attention. But the truth is that it goes a *lot* deeper than that.

For example, training with higher rep ranges also triggers angiogenesis. This creates new blood vessels that supply the muscle with oxygen and nutrients. This is crucial for both muscle recovery and better strength endurance via the supply of metabolites. This can also help to shuttle waste products away from the muscle to reduce fatigue.

Increasing blood supply to various parts of the body is critical for helping rapid recovery from injury and it can lead to much faster muscle growth. I have found this myself: I used to train almost exclusively with high-repetition push-ups. I'd use a fast cadence and short range of motion and maintain "continuous time under tension." This flooded the muscles with blood and made my pecs my most developed feature growing up.

---

54 Troy A. Hornberger & Karyn Esser, "Mechanotransduction and the regulation of protein synthesis in skeletal muscle," *Proceedings of The Nutrition Society* 63, no. 2 (2004): 331–5.

The benefits have followed me throughout my life. I've always been able to bench roughly twice my bodyweight, even during lulls in my training, and I still get compliments on my pec strength. I've never had any injuries there.

The ATG system, spearheaded by Ben Patrick and Keagan Smith that I *highly* recommend, also recommends the use of "pump" style training, or "short range movements" to ensure adequate blood supply to tendons—which have a lesser blood supply and are thus slower to grow and more prone to injury.[55]

Another good reason to increase blood supply is that it helps create satellite cells; studies show a link between capillarization and muscle satellite cell count.[56] Satellite cells live between the basement membrane and plasma membrane of muscle fibers and act like stem cells that can be used to repair and grow skeletal muscle.

And adding more satellite cells and myonuclei also has the benefit of helping us to recover muscle more quickly after a hiatus from training. As far as we know, myonuclei stick around indefinitely after being formed.

This is where we begin to see the merits of varying tempos, rep ranges, and more within our training, too. While someone interested in purely strength might previously have focussed solely on heavy lifts, low rep counts, and muscle damage, we now see that using higher rep ranges to encourage increased blood supply can help *support* that endeavour.

---

55   Keitaro Kubo et al., "Time course of changes in the human Achilles tendon properties and metabolism during training and detraining in vivo," *European Journal of Applied Physiology* 112 (2012): 2679–2691. The study is so nice, I referenced it twice.

56   Indrani Sinha-Hikim et al., "Testosterone-induced muscle hypertrophy is associated with an increase in satellite cell number in healthy, young men," *Am J Physiol Endocrinol Metab* 285, no. 1 (2003):197–205.

Other methods to increase satellite cell count include supplementing with creatine,[57] boosting testosterone, and training with longer training sessions.

Connective Tissue Hypertrophy

What is also important to consider is "connective tissue hypertrophy."

We know that tendons take longer than muscles to grow in response to training due to their lesser blood supply. This is something to keep in mind, seeing how important tendon strength is to overall performance and resilience.

Tendons are capable of withstanding greater tension than muscles. And during activities such as sprinting, they arguably play a larger role.

For these reasons, we may do better to think less in terms of individual muscles and more in terms of "MTUs" or "Muscle Tendon Units."

Beyond that, we should remember that tendons aren't the only type of connective tissue and aren't always so clear-cut and defined. Generally, muscles and tendons connect via special structures called the myotendinous junction and enthesis. These can be thought of as anchor points, but they vary greatly depending on the requirements of the joint.

Aponeuroses are sheets of fibrous tissue that act like large, flat tendons with broad surface areas. This can also be thought of as fascia. But fascia

57   Steen Olsen et al., "Creatine supplementation augments the increase in satellite cell and myonuclei number in human skeletal muscle induced by strength training," *The Journal of Physiology* 573, no. 2 (2006): 525–535.

can also include many other types of tissue. It is best to think of fascia as a cling-film wrap that surrounds the muscles, joints, and organs.

Amazingly, fascia also inserts itself *into* the muscle and divides into pockets called "epimysium." This also protrudes and divides muscle into even more bundles of muscle fibers called fascicles, which are then wrapped in *another* type of connective tissue called perimysium.

This means that connective tissue also contributes to the size and appearance of the muscle! In fact, around 20 percent of muscle is comprised of connective tissue.

Fascia can also contribute to strength by connecting distant muscle groups via "fascial force transmission." This enables many automatic processes critical for our movement and allows for the transmission of signals. For example, when we walk, the heel strike on the right side creates a slight lift in the pelvis to the left. This sudden acceleration is controlled by the contralateral hip abductors, triggering tension across the back that travels up to the opposite latissimus dorsi via the thoracolumbar fascia. Imagine pulling a tight skin over a drum. This is then what causes the opposite arm to swing as we walk, all with zero conscious input from us.[58] A great book for more on this is *Born to Walk* by James Earls.[59]

The fascia helps to maintain the integrity of the entire body as a tensegrity structure. We spoke about this way back in Chapter 1. As a reminder: the body is built like a spiderweb rather than a stack of bones piled on each other like blocks. Fascia maintains the distance between bones and ensures that we can be turned upside down without everything moving around.

---

58   F. H. Willard et al., "The thoracolumbar fascia: anatomy, function and clinical considerations," *Journal of Anatomy* 221, no. 6 (2012): 507–536.

59   You may also be interested in looking up the "spinal engine" to see why some people think this swinging motion is so integral to human movement.

Finally, we know that fascia also contains its own muscle cells, meaning that it can generate its own force. The fascia is plastic and can change via fibroblast cells that lay down collagen and collagenase in response to stress and pressure signals along tension lines. There is much more to learn about the fascia, and it shows how little we still know about how the body can move and generate force.

Training with extreme ranges of motion with high velocity and heavy eccentrics are all methods for training the tendons. Training with a wider variety of movements, particularly outside of the linear patterns we associate with traditional lifting, is the best way to maintain strong and healthy fascia.

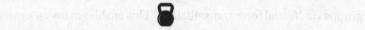

While there's a lot we still don't know, the preceding chapter outlines our best understanding of what makes muscle grow and get stronger.

While moving around more is a powerful stimulus, it won't necessarily involve the necessary mechanical tension, metabolic stress, or muscle damage required to build real muscle. In other words, if we want to be changed by our environment, we need to create a "harsher" environment. Now we have some idea of how to do that.

But this is only scratching the surface of how the body can change in response to training. We hear about muscle damage and metabolic stress, but they're only a small piece of the puzzle.

If we want to go deeper and affect even greater change, we need to look at how the body changes on a neurological and genetic level.

Guess what? That's the topic of the next chapter!

Chapter 9

THE LESSER-KNOWN ADAPTATIONS OF TRAINING

Beyond simply building more muscle and creating thicker muscle fibers, the body can change in several fundamental ways in response to training. By understanding this, we can ensure that our adaptive training program offers the ideal stimulus to tap into those natural transformative capabilities.

We're going deep again; hang on to your hats!

Muscle Fiber Type

Another consideration is muscle fiber type. We have Type 1, Type 2a, and Type 2x muscle fibers that differ in their mitochondria count and ability to express force explosively.

"Slow type" muscle fiber (Type 1) is highly energy efficient and useful for running long distances. Type 1 muscle fibers contain more mitochondria and thus are more aerobic in nature. Fast types (Type 2) contain more ATPase, the enzyme that catalyses ATP from ADP. These muscle types are more "anaerobic."

The truth is that we use both types of muscle fiber during any given exercise and that these fiber types exist along a continuum (rather than as set categories/binaries). It's also true that different muscle groups contain higher densities of fiber types, depending on their typical usage.

Fiber types are also organized into "motor units" comprised of just that type. According to Henneman's size principle, the body will recruit these motor units for any job, starting with the slowest type and adding bigger and more powerful motor units as the goal demands.

We need to know it *is* possible to alter ratios of fiber types within given muscles through training. This is despite claims by those that believe powerlifting is the only true way to improve strength and performance.[60]

Specifically, fiber type is about 50 percent determined by training.[61] Although the changeability of muscle fiber also varies from person to person.

This way, we have another avenue for increasing explosiveness, rate of force development, and even muscle size (seeing as type 2 muscle fiber is thicker than type 1). We do this predominantly by training with explosive movements and ballistic movements. To this end, many people will use plyometric training, which also trains the stretch-shortening cycle (myotatic stretch response) crucial for a lot of athletic performance.

But plyometric nature of this kind, with short ground-contact times, is inferior when stimulating hypertrophy. The low time spent contracted means that metabolic build-up doesn't occur, and the lack of eccentric

---

60 Don't get me started!

61 Ildus Ahmetov et al., "Gene polymorphisms and fiber-type composition of human skeletal muscle," *Int J Sport Nutr Exerc Metab* 22, no. 4 (2012): 292–303; Noriyuki Fuku et al., *Sports, Exercise, and Nutritional Genomics* (Cambridge, MA: Academic Press, 2019), 295–314.

contraction and light weight means not much muscle damage can occur either. Hence, jumping alone won't build massive, tree-trunk legs.

Hormones

Many of these changes are dependent on hormones. I won't go into this in-depth because this has more to do with diet and lifestyle than training, but there are some interesting points to note.

Anabolic hormones like testosterone and growth hormones encourage muscle growth through channels such as the mTOR pathway. mTOR is the mammalian target of rapamycin and is released in response to an increase in energy, nutrients, and protein. In other words: we build more muscle when well-fed, and many of these previous processes depend on that to be effective.

But sarcoplasmic-style training can also further accelerate this effect by encouraging the build-up of substances like lactic acid. Lactic acid has been a scapegoat for the longest time, but it serves many important roles. Not only is lactic acid a key additional fuel for the body but it also stimulates the production of testosterone via Leydig cells.[62] It may also be necessary for growth hormone production.[63] Finally, lactic acid has the effect of drawing water into the muscle to encourage muscle swelling. This may act as a further stimulus for protein synthesis as the tension in the cell is detected.

---

62 H. Lin et al., "Stimulatory effect of lactate on testosterone production by rat Leydig cells," *J Cell Biochem* 83, no 1 (2001):147–54.

63 R. J. Godfrey et al., "The role of lactate in the exercise-induced human growth hormone response: evidence from McArdle disease," *Br J Sports Med* 43, no. 7 (2009): 521–5.

Brain Gains

It's also important to keep in mind the role that the nervous system plays in strength. Pavel Tsatsouline describes strength as a "skill" and, in many cases, he's right.

To utilize the strength of your bicep, you must send a signal to your arm to recruit the corresponding motor units and contract the muscle. See my first book on this.

These motor units correspond with motor neurons in the motor cortex. For example, there are 774 motor units (approximately) in the bicep and the same number of motor neurons for activating them.

However, we cannot activate all these motor units at once for various reasons. What we *can* do, though, is strengthen the signal through training. We do this by causing long-term neuroplasticity in the engrams responsible for particular movement patterns and increasing receptors at the neuromuscular junction.

The former process—cementing the neural pathways responsible for particular movements—is how a martial artist learns to throw an incredibly powerful punch without gaining any muscle. They learn to optimally recruit the motor units necessary to generate the force and become more efficient at relaxing the antagonistic muscle groups that otherwise offer unwanted resistance to slow them down. This is why a powerlifter or bodybuilder can't generate the same force with a punch, despite having far more muscle mass.

In the same way, you can increase your ability to bend steel or perform an ideal bench press.

DNA

But how does all this happen? How does the body know to produce more protein?

That would be due to gene expression, which we touched on in Chapter 1.

DNA is the blueprint for the human body that exists within every cell. It exists multiple times within single muscle cells because a single muscle cell can contain multiple myonuclei.

DNA provides instructions that tell the cell to build proteins. The precise proteins that get built are, in many cases, determined at birth. This is why some of us have blue eyes and some of us have brown eyes.

But it's also possible to alter the expression of DNA by turning on and off specific genes through lifestyle factors such as training and diet. This is the basis for every change within the body, from brain plasticity to protein synthesis to fiber type changes.

We learned earlier about the gene ACTN3 which codes for increased alpha-actinin-3, a protein expressed more so in fast, Type 2 muscle fiber. This is seen more commonly in power-based athletes but there is now some evidence to suggest that supplementing with pequi oil can result in altered gene expression resulting in more transcription for the same.[64]

Moreover, we can increase ACTN3 gene expression through explosive-type training.[65]

---

64   Ieler Ferreira Ribeiro et al., "The influence of erythropoietin (EPO T G) and a-actinin-3 (ACTN3 R577X) polymorphisms on runners' response to the dietary ingestion of antioxidant supplementation based on pequi oil (Caryocar Brasiliense Camb.): a before-after study," *J Nutrigenet Nutrigenomics* 6, no. 6 (2013): 283–304.

65   Daria Domańska-Senderowska et al., "Relationships between the Expression of the ACTN3 Gene and Explosive Power of Soccer Players," *J Hum Kinet* 69 (2019): 79–87.

More evidence that *only* training with one type of training—even powerlifting—won't cut it.

Sorry, it's a whole thing…

So, How Do We Get Stronger?

Okay, so that was quite the infodump.

Sorry!

I feel this was necessary, however, to dispel some of the conveniently simplified explanations of muscle building that back certain approaches to training. The truth is there are *far* too many factors at play here for us to possibly account for all of them. And there are certainly too many different processes for us to rely on a simple training program that only involves *one* type of movement.

A typical powerlifting program leaves so much performance on the table by ignoring strength endurance, blood supply, explosiveness and fiber type, muscle control beyond performance on a few specific lifts, different vectors of movement—including *anything* for the rotational plane…

The same is true for any other training modality.

This was kind of the point of my last book.

(You have read it, haven't you? Buddy?)

Not only should we combine as many different movements as possible, but we should also combine different tempos, volumes, and goals. Again, this would happen *naturally* in a wild environment.

You would not only use the muscle explosively, or only use it for endurance training. You would use it for both. And the results would be superior for long-term health and performance.

You'd walk while tracking prey. Occasionally break into a jog. Then you'd sprint when they got tired, and it was time to close in on them. You might climb a tree, then move a heavy log. Do some wrestling, then squat around the camp and eat.

We can benefit, again, from this kind of variety. For example, someone training purely for strength might use predominantly high-weight/low-rep training. However, we now know that high-rep ranges can improve blood supply to encourage recovery, helping them respond better to training and lift more in the long run.

Plyometric training alone won't give you big arms. But use this training to increase fast twitch fibers and you'll have more potential for size, and more lactate, meaning more anabolic hormone production. Thus, any *subsequent* training may lead to greater growth.

We know that using overcoming isometrics can be a powerful tool for increasing neural drive and muscle fiber recruitment.

If we want greater sarcomeres in series, we need more eccentric training in our lives. But we need more *concentric* training if we want greater sarcomeres in parallel.

We know that rehearsing movements without heavy resistance can improve efficiency, which translates to greater expression of power.

We should consider moving slowly if we want to remove the effect of the strength curve and momentum on our performance and thus gain even greater muscle control.

I am doubling down on everything I said in my first book. One training style is not enough if we want total fitness and performance.

Strength is multifactorial, and so our training must be, too.

That deep dive into muscle and strength building is still woefully shallow and missing a lot of key details. There is still so much we likely don't even know yet.

And that's before I've even spoken about cardio, mobility, or anything else, which are all *just* as complex.

And so, I again suggest what I describe as "Black Box Training." Instead of trying to reverse engineer everything we possibly can about the human body to design the perfect, comprehensive training program, we should instead provide the body with all the stimuli it could expect to receive and "let it do its thing."

The nutritional equivalent would be to stop trying to get every nutrient you read about in a scientific journal and instead aim to eat as *diverse and natural a diet as possible*. Instead of buying thirty pots of supplements, eat lots of vegetables, fruits, and meats. And keep an eye on what the body *evolved* to prefer: organ meats, for example, that contain all those crucial nutrients that fuel the brain and body. And bone, which offers us more collagen and gelatine.

Instead of following one training style—or even creating a single program that aims to incorporate the best of everything, inevitably falling short in some ways—we should aim to move the body in as many different challenging ways as possible, as often as possible, without overtraining.

And this is where more "immersive" training that challenges us to move in countless, dynamic ways in a natural environment becomes extremely powerful.

There are many different schools of thought when it comes to training that aim to "discover" the universal theory of human movement. I'm talking about theories such as GOATA, Functional Patterns, the WeckMethod, etc.

These are all admirable and have a lot to offer. As a nerd about this kind of stuff, I find them fascinating.

But I also think they fail to recognize the sheer complexity of the human body. Or how much there is yet to discover. I believe we cannot decode the body yet and we likely never will. If we do, it will be the result of an advanced AI performing machine learning and then prescribing specific movements and exercises.

The workings of that "theory of everything" will still be alien to us. It will still be a "black box."

Intensity

But if we also want to be "SuperFunctional" then we also need the intensity. That much is clear.

That's where we subtly modify our usual activities to provide more of the key stimuli we have discussed in this chapter, like time under tension, mechanical tension, explosiveness, etc.

As I said before: rock climbing is a perfect example of immersive, black-box training. But to get optimal muscle growth and strength gains from it, we need to tweak our approach so that the goal isn't to get to the top but maintain tension across the lats and forearms, for example.

We can perform rock climbing with a weighted vest. Rock climbing using only the arms to get to the top. Rock climbing where we perform three pull-up reps on every ascent.

We become better at the skill itself by performing it with increased intensity and challenge (this is the SAID principle in a nutshell—Specific Adaptations to Imposed Demands), but we also become *generally* more performant in a way that can transition to other activities.

It's repetition without repetition. Variety with consistency.

ATNSP

There's another way to look at this: which is to say that by training skills, you can train the largest number of attributes and traits.

In my previous book, I introduced the ATSP hierarchy. I have since updated this to be the "ATNSP" hierarchy, which does a better job of accounting for the movement patterns that get laid down as neural maps and fascial connections between muscles.

ATNSP stands for the following:

Attributes

A fundamental physical aspect of a person. For example: strong biceps.
Or, to get even more granular: high fast twitch density in the biceps.

Traits

Traits are slightly more broad concepts that are expressed *by* attributes.
These are things like "strength," "speed," or "endurance." If we see
enough of a certain trait expressed throughout the body, we might go so
far as to describe that person as "having" that trait. We might say a person
is "strong" or "fast."

While some traits might generally be more systemic, such as
cardiovascular fitness, there is no such thing as a truly "global" trait. A
person can have strong pecs and weak calves. Likewise, they might have
greater endurance in their upper body, owing to a lot of rowing, for
example. Blood supply, twitch fiber type, and mitochondria can all affect
endurance in *specific* body parts.

Networks

A network is a combination of attributes often used in conjunction. We
see this most often in particular movement patterns.

For example, the "serape effect" is a twisting motion used when throwing.
This is an important way for the body to generate massive amounts of
power by recruiting the maximum number of motor units. We could
also consider something like the gait cycle to be a network of automatic
movements across the body, as we discussed earlier concerning tensegrity
and the fascial network.

Just as easily, though, we could consider something like the brain's salience network to be a network. This is not a single brain region working by itself but rather a series of interconnected brain regions that appear to "light up" when we are directing our attention in a certain way.[66]

All these rungs on the ladder are open to interpretation as the need demands—this is simply a tool for description and thought. A network can be a simple connection between two muscles or something far more complex.

Skills

Skills are techniques an individual is required to learn. For example, this could be a golf swing, a boxing jab, a dyno in climbing, a perfect deadlift, a handstand, a backflip, a baseball bat swing, or a plie.

Skills are made up of multiple networks, usually working in tandem.

Proficiency

A proficiency is the activity the individual is interested in pursuing. To this end, they need the right attributes, traits, networks, and skills. For example, if they want to learn football (soccer), they will benefit from learning to kick, dribble, header the ball, sprint, jog, tackle, etc.

---

66 Vinod Menon & Lucina Q. Uddin, "Saliency, switching, attention and control: a network model of insula function" *Brain Struct Funct* 214, no. 5–6 (2010): 655–667.

Applying the ATNSP Hierarchy

I use the ATNSP hierarchy when training people to identify the best exercises to achieve a specific goal. The aim is to train at every level so that we build strong and endurant muscles with great control; we build the connections between those muscles into powerful networks, and we practice the skills and proficiency to put those things into practice.

For example, if someone needs to get better at javelin, we can identify they are using the serape effect to some degree. We can then identify the muscles they need to train to become more powerful in that range: the rhomboids, serratus anterior, and internal and external obliques. They also need, of course, to train the glutes, shoulders, and lats. We can train these muscles individually with the Russian twist, bent-over rows, etc. Then we can train the network with cable wood choppers, sledgehammer tire slams, and rotational med ball slams.

But then we *also* need to train the skills and the proficiencies. We need to rehearse the movement patterns (practice that basketball dribble over and over) and utilize them in a real competitive setting. The latter is crucial to enjoying things like the interference effect and all that chaotic disorganization—the repetition without repetition that comes from real-world practice outside a controlled setting.

Yes, the proficiency must be trained as well. This is the missing ingredient for those that train purely *to train*. And it's why our fitness is often lacking.

Proficiency can also refer to our ability in daily waking life and all the little tasks that encompasses.

The problem with most modern fitness is that we train the attributes and traits to the detriment of everything else. And as we can see, they are relatively useless on their own. A strong bicep is great, but it can't do much if it's attached to a weak shoulder and grip or if you haven't practiced using it for carrying or pull-ups.

Our training is isolated, clinical, and repetitive—everything that the real world is not.

We're flipping that on its head. We're taking the proficiencies—such as sports, swimming, climbing, and trail running—and using that to train the maximum number of attributes, traits, and networks. At least, that is part of what we're doing.

And we're training with exercise flows and combinations (Vector Sets) that naturally incorporate many elements.

Intensity and Optimal Performance

The levels of the ATNSP hierarchy work both ways. Train the attributes and you will inevitably improve the skills. Train the skills and you will train the attributes. But there is a "trickle down" effect, where the benefits become less the more rungs removed.

Playing football will only strengthen your quads so much. Leg extensions will only improve your football game *so much*.

The thing is, were we to train at just one level, it should be the top: the skills. Because this is what we need, after all, and this will result in the widest variety of attributes, traits, and skills.

Training programs fail to make us healthier in many cases because they miss so many crucial aspects of our ability. What training program can you possibly think of that trains all the strength and performance you expect, along with mobility across the body, grip strength, rotational strength, single leg strength, balance, straight arm strength, situational awareness, sports vision, impulse control, endurance, VO2 max, lung strung, focus, toe strength, tibialis anterior, quadratus lumborum, an ideal gait cycle, coordination?

I have given it my best shot with **SuperFunctional Training 2.0: The Protean Performance System**, which you can find on my website.

But that's a complex training program that still misses some of these points.

It's simply impossible to train everything by taking this reductionist approach.

I am no minimalist. I am a maximalist. We maximalists have been subdued long enough; it's time we make a comeback!

I do not believe in Occam's Razor. I don't understand the desire to reduce all the incredible complexity around us to a few simple rules.

Isn't it more likely that the incredible complexity all around us is the result of *lots* of *extremely* complex rules?

Thus, we must train the skills and the proficiencies we want and then see the performance across the board. We pick up all those fundamental human movements, train obscure things like ankle strength, and keep our brains engaged and working the entire time.

But if we want to be SuperFunctional, we not only need to engage in a comprehensive suite of highly dynamic and chaotic activities; we must also perform these in a way that will trigger a change in the human body.

We need those stimuli: muscle damage, learning, varied movement, metabolic stress, and mechanical tension. And we need to train with enough frequency and intensity to force adaptation if we want to go beyond "healthy."

There are a few ways to go about this, depending on what is the most practical for you.

1. Engage in a range of sports, hobbies, or activities that provide a wide range of useful attributes and traits. Increase the difficulty, forget the usual goals, and *make* this training with a focus on muscle damage, metabolic stress, etc. Not every activity is made equal for this purpose. For example, football or wrestling are fantastic options. Rowing is a lot more repetitive and linear. I will refer to the "right" type of activities as **"Dynamic Activities."** And by increasing the intensity, we are engaging in **"High-Intensity Dynamic Activity Training."**

2. Invent new activities, sports, and hobbies specifically designed to trigger maximum adaptation. For example, use the two-person training games in the next chapter. Again, keep the pressure on to trigger that change. This is an example of High-Intensity Dynamic Activity Training.

3. Make training *more like* the involved, dynamic activities we've discussed and would have engaged in during our evolution. That means spreading training throughout the day or breaking it into chunks (**Modular Training**), using a wider variety of movements and avoiding rote repetition, and increasing the cognitive element to become more engaged. Perhaps training outside to introduce more chaotic elements. I shall refer to this going forward as **Chaos Training**.

You may recall the **Slow and Mechanically DisAdvantaged Movement Training** (SANDAM) that I discussed in the last book. This was my first stab at more dynamic "Black Box" training that could be brought to the gym. You may also have encountered **Gauntlet Sets** from SuperFunctional 2.0, which utilize multiple movements in a more organized fashion. These are good options, but I am now also recommending **Vector Sets**. Vector Sets are another example of Chaos Training.

Simply training outside is another simple way to make training more chaotic. You can perform the same calisthenics routine or cardio circuit but use grass and trees instead of flat ground. Likewise, training with tools like kettlebells, sandbags, med balls, etc., will make your training more chaotic.

4. Make your environment and habit naturally more challenging so you are constantly being trained by your routine. Do this with **Incidental Training** and with smart changes to your environment. The latter I call **Adaptive Immersion Training**. This way, you can lower the intensity while increasing frequency.

Don't think of training as binary. Don't think of either training or *not* training. Think about to what *extent* your current activity is training you. And what is it training?

Of course, you can also combine or mix and match these.

This is adaptive training.

For example, my current training program consists of:

*   Lots of punches and kicks performed against a heavy bag *or* shadowboxing (**High-Intensity Dynamic Activity Training**).

*   Learning to juggle while on the balance board (**High-Intensity Dynamic Activity Training**). Neither of these activities is done

during "workouts" but rather when it takes my fancy. I also go trail running.

- Training toward several advanced calisthenics movements. I've split the upper body routine into a push in the morning and pull in the evening, and I perform the mobility portion even later, thus making it **Modular Training**.

   I also incorporate traditional strength training and kettlebell training as part of the same workouts.

- Once a week I film outside and make a point to make it a stimulating workout, too. This involves throwing medicine balls, climbing trees, walking on my hands, performing **Vector Sets** of push-ups and handsprings on the uneven grass, kettlebell swings, etc.—**Chaos Training**.

- I use **Incidental Training** throughout the day. I practiced a handstand a minute ago and did pistol squats holding my daughter this morning.

Our environment and our habits are what shape our bodies predominantly. Our lives.

We need more life. *Harder.*

In the next chapter, you'll see how you can develop your adaptive training routine.

Chapter 10

YOUR ADAPTIVE TRAINING ROUTINE

We've covered a lot of theory at this point, and I promised this book would have actual, practical takeaways.

Well, I am a man of my word. In this chapter you'll find adjustments you can make to your everyday life that will help you to get stronger and more mobile by "osmosis" simply by existing in your environment. You will find fitness games and activities you can engage in to get stronger while having fun.

You will find a full, adaptive training routine.

And you will find an option for training *without* training—performing a series of activities and hobbies that will take care of your fitness and make you highly performant.

Let's get to it.[67]

Adaptive Training = Incidental Training, Chaos Training, Adaptive Immersion Training, Modular Training, Vector Sets, High-Intensity Dynamic Activity Training

---

67 Note that this chapter will not contain exercise descriptions. That is beyond the scope of this already-pretty-long book. Fortunately, these are easy enough to find and many of them have been discussed on my *Bioneer* YouTube channel.

Incidental Training Protocol

Here are some suggestions for training throughout the day. By harnessing naturally occurring opportunities to train, you can work on aspects of your performance that you might otherwise neglect.

Horse Stance While Brushing Teeth

Horse stance (mabu) is a wide stance from Kung Fu that builds deep core muscles along with greater hip flexibility. Many of us lack ideal hip mobility, making this a great choice for a form of incidental training. If you brush your teeth for two to three minutes, this is a great amount of time. As it gets easier, widen the stance.

It's even possible to reach a full middle-split using this method.[68] FitnessFAQs has an excellent video on this topic.

Left-Handed Toothbrushing

Left-handed toothbrushing is a fun little challenge for your motor control.

One Hundred Calf Raises

Another great option while brushing your teeth is performing one hundred calf raises. It is said that performing a hundred daily calf raises can be an effective method to overcome plateaus in the calves and force

---

68   It's on my to-do list.

some hypertrophy. I perform calf raises when brushing my teeth at night and horse stance when brushing them in the morning.

Heel Walk

Walk on your heels to train the tibialis anterior.

Grip Training

Grip training can be performed anywhere. I keep a grip trainer by my kettle and do this while the kettle boils.

Chair L-Sits

Every time you sit in a chair, raise your legs into an L-sit and hold to failure. Okay, maybe not every time. This is not particularly appropriate at a funeral, for example. That goes for most of these things.

Overcoming Isometric Crunch

Another option for training while seated is to place your hands on your knees and then try and force your torso so that your chest touches your legs. Hold with effort.

Toe Pushes

Push your toes into the ground with force to train them.

No one can see this exercise. Meaning you kind of *could* do it at a funeral? That's up to you, though.

Forward Lean

When bored standing, try leaning gently forward until you use your toes to keep yourself upright.

Mental Math/Mini-Meditation

When standing in a queue, going down an escalator, or otherwise doing something dull, try and perform mental math. I recommend a problem that includes a big cognitive load, such as multiplying two large numbers that will force lots of "carrying over" and can't rely on memorized patterns.

In my previous book, I discussed how many of the benefits of meditation are a result of the intense focus required. Mental math can offer some of these same benefits.[69] That said, a quick "mini-meditation" can also be effective.

Stair Bounding

The day you stop taking the stairs three at a time is the day you begin your journey to not being able to. If you've given up this little form of expression, consider taking it up again.

---

69 Matthew A. Scult et al., "Thinking and Feeling: Individual Differences in Habitual Emotion Regulation and Stress-Related Mood Are Associated with Prefrontal Executive Control," *Psychological Science* 5, no. 1 (2016): 150–157.

Squatting

Any time you drop something on the floor, perform a deep squat to pick it up. This is also how my daughter climbs on and dismounts when carrying her. A nice sixteen-kilogram front squat!

I also deep squat when I fill the tyres with air. When I change my son's nappy. When I need to check my phone and it's plugged in on the floor…

Carries

Loaded carries are one of the best forms of exercise because they straddle that line between exercise and activity. They are chaotic in nature and train multiple traits and attributes.

Going to the car? Why not bring your kettlebell with you?

Or even keep your kettlebell by the stairs and carry it up and down every time you travel that way.

Doorway Pull-Up Bar

The old classic example of greasing the groove. Keep a pull-up bar in your doorway and blast out three clean reps every time you pass through.

Verbal Fluency Practice

If you're reading something, why not read it aloud and try to perform it as well as you can? This is a great way to practice your speech and verbal fluency and a great example of how you can turn anything into training simply by *trying your hardest*. It becomes training as soon as you increase the effort and attention.

What else can you try to do as well as possible each time you do it? Even being mindful of your walking gait and trying to improve it, possibly with some background reading, is a great example. Bringing more awareness to your movement and improving a technique you'll use every day.

Straddle Sit

Watching TV? Why not start with a deep straddle sit? The same goes for any form of mobility.

Light Switch with Foot

If you need to turn on the light switch and are physically able, try doing it with your foot. I try and use a slow, controlled sidekick. This trains balance, mobility, and end-range strength all at once. Though I often get a cramp.

Foot Pick Up

Any time I pick up something soft, I do it with my feet. That means socks, children's cuddly toys, etc. Everything in my house, presumably, smells of foot.

"Opportunities to Move"

I keep little opportunities and reminders to move around my home and office. My living room has a yoga wheel and parallettes. I'll often stop what I'm doing to do a handstand. I also have juggling balls and a Rubik's cube in here.

There's also a balance beam that comes out from time to time.

My garden has a pull-up bar attached to the wall with a rope and a kettlebell that lives outside.

My kitchen has a grip trainer and another kettlebell.

But my office, where it is all too easy to sit for long periods, has dip bars, a balance board, another kettlebell, more juggling balls, dumbbells, a weight bench, and more. I have a free-standing pull-up bar in the post. I feel like a kid entering this room. The first thing I want to do is to hang from the dip bars or balance on my board.

Remove Opportunities to *Not* Move

You can also take the opposite approach. For example, my friend and collaborator Liam Ellis has removed all furniture from his home, forcing himself to sit on the floor. This is excellent for posture, mobility, and more.

He also goes barefoot into cafes and around town. He's a little more hardcore than me and has that luxury owing to the lack of cohabiting three-year-olds.

But if you want to enjoy even greater benefits, this is the next step. Heck, I'd even recommend keeping belongings you regularly need on the floor (again, as long as you don't have a kid or dog that will eat them) and squatting over the toilet.

To begin implementing incidental training, I'd recommend choosing two or three. Then incorporate more into your lifestyle once those are deep-set.

Horse stance toothbrushing and grip training during the kettle-boil offer an easy place to start.

Fitness Games

Fitness games are an example of highly dynamic and unpredictable **High-Intensity Dynamic Activity Training**. That's thanks to the hugely unpredictable nature of other people.

Depending on what kind of mates you have…

Balance Beam Battle

This one has a high risk of injury, so practice with caution. Simply square off against an opponent while standing on a railing or similar, then attempt to push one another off. The last one standing is the winner.

This can be performed crawling, which makes for a more core and grip-intensive workout, or standing, which is more of a balance challenge.

Bunny Hop Battle

We used to do this at karate, though I've made up the name. Basically, we all squat on the balls of our feet and bounce around the dojo, trying to push each other over. You could only get around by doing short bunny hops. It's great training for the knees (if they're up to it), good cardio, and a balance challenge, too.

Piggy-Back Battle

We used to play this at school when the field was open. There were only a few (hundred) minor (and major) injuries.

You need at least four people for this one. Each team consists of someone on the bottom and someone on top—on the other person's shoulders. The objective was to try and push the other person off the top.

Actually, I don't recommend this. This is a recipe for a serious injury. What the heck were we thinking?

Wrestling

Simply wrestling with a friend is one of the best exercises you can enjoy. You don't need to know Jujitsu to benefit from this, either. Just make some ground rules, then try and get each other to the ground.

Sparring

Similarly, sparring is a fantastic option for training cardio, improving reflexes, developing techniques, and more. This can be done as no-contact or touch-sparring.

You'll be surprised how exhausting this is, but it's also great for your focus and mental endurance.

Rage Froobling

Rage Froobling is a strange combination between wrestling and parkour (free running). The name comes from the video that perhaps created the idea (maybe?), Teghead. It was recently featured in a video by JimmyTheGiant.

The idea is simple: two challengers attempt to climb a wall before the other can. The twist is that they can also try and pull each other off/wrestle. They can also block each other or grapple each other to prevent them from trying to climb the wall.

Again, this could be risky, so practice with caution!

Lizard Crawl Tag

Like it sounds: play tag, except you need to lizard crawl instead of running.

Of course, regular tag is also an option.

Partner Kettlebell Juggling

This requires a lot of practice and training before it should be attempted. It's awesome to behold, though—check it out on YouTube.

Tug of War

All you need is a friend and a rope. Play the best out of ten and see how tired your grip is at the end and how out of breath you are.

Med Ball Catch

A simpler option would be a game of catch using a med ball. Start light and go gentle.

Nathan's Crazy Pec Blast

My friend Nathan created this exercise when we were at uni together. I knew it was awesome then and all my research since has only confirmed this.

One person lies on the bench holding two moderately heavy dumbbells. A partner stands over them and then uses their hands and instructions to guide them through the movements. For example, Nathan would tell me:

"Dumbbell press! Dumbbell press! Left arm only! Right arm only! Press to halfway and hold! Keep holding, keep holding! Dumbbell press! Dumbbell fly! Dumbbell fly! Push against my hands! Keep pushing!"

And so forth. Then it would be my go. It's fun and challenging and it led to some crazy pec growth. Of course, the same thing can be done on a pull-up bar or anything else.

Notice that this is basically a **Vector Set!**

Follow the Leader

A fairer way to do this kind of training, which doesn't invite quite the same levels of sadism, is to have the partner perform the exercise and the other person attempt to copy it. An ideal situation would be to have two pull-up bars opposite each other. One person leads, and the other attempts to follow. Rest and swap roles.

Activities for a Perfectly Rounded Physique and Performance

Many dynamic activities, sports, and hobbies can forge an incredibly well-rounded performance profile.

For example, one combination that would make most people SuperFunctional by any measure:

- Kickboxing
- Rock climbing
- Yoga

Or how about:

- Dance

- Jujitsu

- Piano

Or:

- Trail running

- Swimming

- Gymnastics

Or:

- Football

- Aerial arts

- Boxing

Or (perhaps for an older demographic):

- Hiking

- Badminton

- Juggling

These activities combined will develop amazing strength, endurance, mobility, balance, coordination, and general health for almost anyone. They're fun and social, and there's no need to step foot inside a "gym" or perform a "workout."

Perform them with greater intensity and focus to benefit from High-Intensity Dynamic Activity Training.

Increasing Intensity

So, what can you do to increase the intensity?

Some properties we're looking to accentuate are continuous time under tension (maintaining pressure on one muscle group to induce fatigue and promote metabolic stress), mechanical tension, and muscle damage.

Repetition without Repetition

Let's say you're bouldering—rock climbing without a rope. To make this a better stimulus for muscle growth, you can repeat each move five times as you ascend the wall. For example: climb to the top of the climbing wall, but each time you pull or push yourself up, lower yourself again, and repeat. Maintain tension in the working muscles the entire time.

The same thing works for parkour: design a short sequence but include repetitions as you complete it. For example: do three climb-ups instead of one, drop back down each time, do some muscle-ups before your lache. Do a precision to a beam, squat on the beam several times, then spring off.

We can also create drills of similar movements. For boxing, for example, hit the bag with techniques using the back hand repeatedly until fatigued, then swap sides.

In dance, you can design a dance that utilizes high reps of some of the more physically challenging movements strung together.

Pre-Fatigue

Pre-fatiguing a muscle is a technique from bodybuilding that usually involves tiring the supporting muscle groups to force the primary muscles to work harder during an exercise.

We're going to use it a little differently here by training all the muscles that are used for an activity so that the subsequent activity is more likely to create muscle damage and stimulate growth.

For example, if you were going to do some rock climbing, you could first do a session of lat pull-downs and chin-ups, maybe with some squats and grip training for good measure. Now do your rock climbing and feel the burn.

Cardio Acceleration

Training with a cool name!

This technique involves cardio between sets to maintain a high heartrate throughout an entire workout.

As you can guess, we're applying this same strategy to other forms of training. For example, if you were playing football with friends, you could make the rule for yourself that you will run *the entire time*. While waiting for the ball, you will be jogging on the spot.

Or you could do some cardio prior to your sparring to pre-fatigue yourself. This is also extremely beneficial for improving mental vigilance. Can you still focus when tired and stressed out?

Overspeed Training

Perform the usual movements but attempt to be faster to build explosiveness and increase the endurance challenge.

My friend and contributor, Grant Stevens, describes how he applies this idea to his martial arts. To become faster at delivering blows and kicks, he says to focus on *going faster*. It sounds obvious, yet it's something so many forget to do.

How *quickly* can you climb to the top of that climbing wall? How quickly can you perform that dance choreography?

Added Resistance

Perform your usual activity but under weighted conditions. Rock climbing, of course, lends itself well to this. You can also spar with a weight vest, just like Goku. Or how about swimming while tied to something heavy?

How about trying to dance while under a heavy load? Or even while carrying a kettlebell? How do you look graceful while doing this?

Be careful to avoid injury—start light. Consider, too, how this added weight might alter your technique negatively. It's to be employed sparingly.

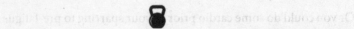

These are some ideas for ways to make your activities more challenging in specific ways that will force rapid adaptation. You'll be training for *truly*

comprehensive performance while simultaneously getting much better at the sport or activity in question.

Adaptive Training Routine

Here is a modular training routine that utilizes Vector Sets and chaotic elements to create a well-rounded performance.

Note the way that I have written out the Vector Sets. You have a main exercise, followed by a "pool" of exercises that you can select from. Your objective is to perform fifteen repetitions without rest, alternating between these different examples.

You can do this with a call and response system if you have a partner. You can record instructions for yourself prior. Or, best of all, you can be creative and ad-lib.

Find that it's a bit mentally taxing trying to think of the next exercise while also counting reps and performing the movements? Find yourself getting confused or lacking inspiration?

Good.

Rest for one minute between sets.

Of course, you may add to the exercises in the pool or ignore those you can't do. Complete movements in a controlled manner and make sure you practice everything in an isolated fashion before attempting it as part of a set.

For a warm-up, I highly recommend shadowboxing with a combination of kicks and punches. You can also try skipping or bouncing and catching a reaction ball against a wall to practice coordination.

Then start with lighter versions and easier variations to ease yourself into the correct movement patterns.

Then go to town.

Day One: Upper Body

Module One: Push

3 x 15 Push-Ups (Push-Ups, Archer Push-Up, Lizard Crawl, Isometric Hold, Slow Tempo, Explosive Push-Up, One Arm Push-Up, Wide Push-Up, Narrow Push-Up, Knuckle Push-Up)

3 x 10 Pike Push-Ups (Pike Push-Ups, Slow, Hindu Push-Ups, Downward Dog Hold, Press to Handstand, Handstand Press Up)

Module Two: Pull

3 x 8 Pull-Ups (Pull-Up, Chin-Up, Headbanger, Around the World, Chin-Up Hold, Pull-Up Hold, One Arm Pull-Up/Chin-Up, Assisted One Arm, Explosive Pull-Up, Slow Negative, Arched Back Pull-Up, Tactical Pull-Up, Typewriter Pull-Up)

3 x 10 Bodyweight Rows (Bodyweight Row, Scapula Row, Tuck Front Lever Hold, One Arm Row, Row Hold, Single Arm Row with a Twist)

Module Three: Mobility

2 x 1 Minute Hang

2 x 3 Slow Skin the Cat

Day Two: Lower Body

Module One: Glutes and Hams

3 x 15 Squats (Squats, Sumo Squat, Jump Squat, Isometric Hold, Slow Quasi-Isometric, Pistol Squat, Hindu Squat, Split Squat, Squat Front Kick, Deep Squat, Scissor Jump Squat)

3 x 10 Kettlebell Swings (Kettlebell Swing, Kettlebell Sports Swing, One Arm Swing, Kettlebell Swing Into Squat, Kettlebell Swing Into Snatch, Kettlebell Swing Into Kneeling Snatch, Kettlebell Overhead Squat, Atlas Swing[70])

Module Two: Quads and Back

3 x 10 Hindu Squats (Hindu Squat, Sissy Squat, Sissy Squat Hold, Bunny Hops, Pehalwani Baithak,[71] Kazotsky Kick/Squat Kick)

2 x 8 Back Bridges (Back Bridge, Half Bridge, Glute Bridge, Single Leg Glute Bridge, Tabletop, Crab Crawl, Crab Reach[72])

---

70 It is important that you feel comfortable with all these techniques before attempting to create sequences like this. Kettlebell swings are highly technical with a high injury risk.

71 Pehalwani Baithak is a Hindu Squat with a slight backward jump.

72 Include holds, but don't perform these explosively.

Module Three: Mobility

2 x 1 Minute Spider-Man Stretch

2 x 1 Minute Deep Squat

2 x 1 Minute Straddle Stretch

Day Three: Full Body

Module One: Upper Body Transitions

2 x 10 Burpees (Burpees, Single Leg Burpees, Push-Ups, Squats, Squat Jumps, 100-Up Major, Kick Through)

2 x 10 Muscle Ups (Muscle Up, Pull-Up, Bar Dip, Explosive Pull-Up, Slow Tempo)

Module Two: Twists and Integration

2 x 10 Cable/Band Punch Out (Cable Punch Out, One Arm Cable Press)

2 x 15 Total (Push-Up, Explosive Push-Up, One Arm Push-Up, Kickthrough, Lizard Crawl, Bear Crawl, Lateral Step Push-Up, Burpee, One Leg Burpee, Squat, Jump Squat, Scissor Jump Squat, Deep Squat, Hindu Squat, Sissy Squat, Squat Kick)

Module Three: Core

2 x 10 Hanging Leg Raises (Hanging Leg Raises, Toes to Bar, Frog Kicks, Swings, Hanging Around the Worlds, L-Sit)

2 x 10 Plank (Plank, LaLanne Push-Up Hold, Plank Walk Outs, Side Plank, Reverse Plank, Tabletop, Crab Reach, Lateral Plank Walk, Bird Dog)

Day Four: Rest

Day Five: Upper Body

Module One: Push

3 x 8 Pseudo Planche Push-Ups (Pseudo Planche Push-Up, Pseudo Planche Lean, Tuck Planche Hold)

3 x 8 Dips (Dips, L-Sit Hold, Tuck Planche Dips)

3 x 15 Crazy Pec Fly (Dumbbell Press, Pec Fly, One Arm Dumbbell Press, Holds, Slows, DB Around the World, Overcoming Isometric Press[73])

---

73   The last is only workable with a partner.

Module Two: Pull

3 x 15 Alternating Dumbbell Curls (Alternating Dumbbell Curls, Bilateral DB Curl, Hammer Curl, Drag Curl, Cheat Hammer Curl, Zottman Curl, Holds)

3 x 15 Renegade Rows (Renegade Row, Renegade Row with a Twist, Man Makers, Devil Press, Weighted Crawl, Bent Row)

Module Three: Mobility

2 x 1 Minute Bridge/Half Bridge

2 x 1 Minute Hang

2 x 1 Minute Deep Squat

Day Six Lower Body

Module One: Athleticism

2 x 50 Lunge Walks (Lunge Walk, Squat Walk, Bunny Hops, Lateral Squat Walk, Roll)

2 x 15 Dumbbell Squats (Dumbbell Squat, Dumbbell Jump Squat, Overhead Dumbbell Squat, Dumbbell Clean and Press, Devil Press)

Module Two: Frontal Plane and Core

2 x 8 Dumbbell Romanian Deadlifts (DB Romanian Deadlift, Straight Leg Deadlift, Contralateral Single Leg Romanian Deadlift, Ipsilateral Single Leg Romanian Deadlift, Single Leg Bodyweight Romanian Deadlift, Anterior Reach, Bodyweight Good Morning)

2 x 15 Cossack Squats (Cossack Squat, Side Squat, Lateral Squat Walk)

Module Three: Mobility

2 x 1 Minute Spider-Man Stretch

2 x 1 Minute Deep Squat

2 x 1 Minute Straddle Stretch

Day Seven Rest

If you struggle to ad-lib these movements or create the right stimulus for yourself, visit my website and head to the shop where you'll find **Vector Workouts**. This is a sequence of files containing lots of different sequences for varying ability levels, set to cool music. There's also a "random generator" app and tool to make your own.

Or, at least, I think it's cool.

Of course, you can also alter the split and train fewer times per week if needed.

A Full Body Outdoor Workout

Below is an example outdoor workout that trains the entire body. (You can use Vector Set varieties for these if you prefer.)

- 10 minutes Trail Running
- 2 x 8 Tree Branch Pull-Ups
- 2 x 8 Tree Branch Chin-Ups
- 2 x 20 Push-Ups OR 2 x 12 Branch Dips
- 2 x 8 Pike Push-Ups (Use a Bench or Log)
- 2 x 8 Overhead Log Presses OR 2 x 8 Log Landmine Presses
- 2 x 8 Elevated Pistol Squats
- 2 x 15 Lunge Walks with Log on Shoulders (Each Step is a Rep)
- Superset: 2 x 15 Goblet Squats | 2 x 15 Hindu Squats
- 2 x 8 Cossack Squats
- 2 x 8 Hanging Leg Raises OR 2 x 5 Dragon Flags[74]
- 2 x 15 Rock Piles[75]
- 2 x 8 Glute Bridges
- 2 x 5 Reverse Hypers with Hold

There are countless more options out there and I don't see any difficulty with training outside. If it sounds like I'm trying to convince you, it's because a lot of commenters seem to think it's not possible or impractical. Even if you live in an urban area or park, a single tree can do the trick.

Use your environment and be creative. And for bonus points, bring a med ball, sandbag, or kettlebell with you—even some gymnastic rings.

---

74 Use a park bench.

75 Move a rock or log from the ground on your left to the right and then reverse and repeat. This is essentially a twisting deadlift performed with light weight for reps.

Chapter 11

YOU ARE INFORMATION

They say you should write every book as if it were your last. To that end, I'd like to indulge myself for a moment by exploring a little of the philosophy underpinning this book. Below, you will find no practical advice: only speculation on the nature of life and the future of training.

It gets nerdy. You have been warned.

If you take one thing from this book, it should be that you are a product of your environment.

All training is a hack. The body is not intended to adapt to training; rather it is intended to adapt to the lifestyle demands placed upon it. The best training, therefore, is training that is integrated into our lifestyles and designed to mimic how we are affected by the world around us.

And this doesn't just apply to training. I believe it applies to every aspect of our physicality and psychology.

For example: the best way to learn a language, as I pointed out earlier, is through immersion. You simply immerse yourself in another country and culture, and your brain's natural plasticity will do the rest. You'll unconsciously make connections through the repeated, gentle exposure.

I believe virtual reality will be the key to unlocking truly incredible human performance. When we can immerse ourselves in an environment that challenges us to stay completely aware and move our entire bodies in challenging and novel ways…

When that virtual environment gamifies the experience to make it inherently fun. And when machine learning and computer vision combine to provide real-time feedback, sensitive to minute differences in posture and alignment…

We'll be able to mould our bodies and minds into the best they can be.

And I think the mind will house the most untapped potential. Whether it's regaining a near-photographic working memory or even altering our language to something that allows us to process information *faster*. Or whether it's improving our movement efficiency.

This is the way to a Transhuman-like experience, in my opinion. Not prosthetics and genetic manipulation that, once again, drastically overestimate our understanding of the human body.

It's not transhumanism or posthumanism at all. It's MaxHumanism! Maximizing what's already there beyond what we currently think possible.

And again, we're doing this by changing the environment. The trick is, with virtual reality, we have unlimited control over said environment and how we interact with it.

That's my hot take, anyway. And why I believe fitness truly must be the major selling point for VR.

When a device is light enough to allow for training without lots of sweat and discomfort, when it tracks hands and feet, and when it can incorporate objects from the environment—such as training tools—I think we'll see rapid adoption (with the right software).

For now, we have adaptive training.

You Were Crafted by the Environment

Likewise, if we ever wanted to create artificial intelligence, I believe the only way we could do it would be by creating a virtual environment first.

While there are attempts at recreating neural maps in a simulated environment that seem impressive on the surface, they are severely lacking in terms of their complexity.

IBM's Blue Brain project has run some incredible simulations. On one occasion, it even ran an artificial neural network that simulated half a mouse's brain! In 2013, researchers from Japan and Germany managed to simulate 1 percent of the human brain, modelling a network of an incredible 1.73 billion nerve cells and 10.4 trillion synapses, running on the K Computer (the fourth fastest supercomputer in the world, at that time).[76]

This has led to claims by many entrepreneurs that we are on the brink of creating human-like intelligence.

But the human brain is *far* more than a mere network of neurons.

---

76 Much of this comes from the book *Crux* by Ramez Naam.

As we've seen, the human brain is in a constant state of fluctuation. New neural connections are being formed all the time. As we've seen, this may even be an underlying mechanism of working memory—giving us our ability to think.

We do not understand the rules of plasticity nearly well enough to model this. We've discussed and admitted that we don't *know* if this is how working memory even operates. We don't know which conditions should favour a new connection or not. We don't understand how all the neurotransmitters act on these connections. There are likely *many* more neurotransmitters to discover.

We don't fully understand the role of glial cells. These white cells outnumber the better-known grey brain cells and appear to serve critical roles in maintaining and supporting the actions of neurons. They have not been included in any brain scans or artificial neural networks thus far.

Nor do scans of neural networks consider the effects of "short-term plasticity" that can make neurons more or less likely to fire. They don't understand how double-stranded DNA breakages might be fundamental to supporting rapid brain plasticity…

Even if we had a powerful enough computer to perfectly copy the human brain, we'd never be able to program the laws underpinning it. It would be a static "snapshot" of a brain, at best. Unable, perhaps, to change its mind. To experience different moods. To manipulate information.

It would not be alive.

We are a million miles from anything close to human thought in a simulated environment, and the likes of Elon Musk, who believe otherwise, are mistaken (or, perhaps, intentionally misleading).

Just my humble opinion.

Moreover, attempts at simulating human thought miss that thought
is *inextricably* linked to movement and the physical body, as
discussed earlier.

This is true on a basic level. For example, our moods and thoughts are, to
a large extent, influenced by our guts. Neurotransmitters and hormones
are created outside the brain by gut bacteria and several other organs.

But it goes much deeper.

In my previous book, I discussed the concept of "embodied cognition."
This is a theory that explains how intelligent thought likely arises from
interactions with a physical environment.

When someone tells us about their walk through the woods, we likely
understand it by relating that to our experiences of walking through the
woods. Whether that's by visualizing what they're saying, by feeling the
sensation of the wind on our skin... When listening to these kinds of
stories, areas of the brain light up as though they were happening to us.

Moreover, our abstract understanding of the world is built on this
foundation. We understand quantities because we have experienced
multiple objects in our environment. We understand speed and
relativity and everything else that allows complex thought only due to a
development founded in a physical environment.

To create a "disembodied" intelligence would be to create a being devoid
of goals, meaning, or foundational knowledge. It would not be life as
we know it.

We Are Created by Our Environment

I therefore believe that, to create an artificial being, you would also need to create an artificial environment for them to explore. Moreover, you would need them to learn and grow through their interactions with this artificial environment.

Of course, it needn't look anything like the world we know. It could be a series of numbers on a spreadsheet with no graphical representation. The "intelligence" is essentially an algorithm to compute these other numbers representing the distance and shape of objects.

And, perhaps, that's what our experience could boil down to.

We see contrast and colour as a kind of "shorthand" that allows us to move through the world around us. But all that is, is information.

The problem still exists, though. How would we create this being in the first place to interpret all that information? How do we crack that algorithm?

The answer, I believe, would be through Black Box Training. We would have to create the conditions and allow life to emerge naturally *from* the environment.

Sounds insane? The best way to explain this is with mathematician John Conway's game *Life*.

Life

John Conway's *Life* is a fascinating example of "cellular automation." It was created in 1970 and began life not on a computer but rather on pen and paper.

The idea is simple: you draw a grid with some randomly placed "cells." Then, every "turn," you add or remove cells, based on simple rules. Each turn is called a "generation."

In this case, the rules are:

- A cell with two or more neighbouring cells will survive, unchanged, to the next generation

- A cell with fewer than two neighbours will die (supposed to represent "underpopulation")

- A cell with more than three neighbours dies (representing "overpopulation")

- Empty cells with three live neighbours become live cells (reproduction)

Enter these rules into a computer and create a large enough grid with the right number of starting cells (the initial "seed"), and you'll be treated to a stunning dance of cells that appear to move and swarm around the screen.

Some of the behaviours of these cells can be surprising, however. This is especially true given the simple rules that govern the behaviours.

Over time, common patterns start to form. These include "oscillators" that fluctuate between two or more shapes and survive for many generations (until struck by another "life form"). Then there are the likes of "Blinkers," which appear like rotating rows of three cells. More complex are the "pentadecathlons," which form a variety of circular patterns for fifteen generations before restarting the cycle.

Spaceships are more interesting still: these are structures capable of travelling across the screen. The most common is the arrow-like "Glider."

Then you have "guns" that can launch projectiles across the screen or produce gliders.

Some creations are even capable of "self-replication." These are "lifeforms" capable of creating exact copies of themselves.

This might seem amazing at first, but it is, in fact, inevitable. The same rules of evolution and "survival of the fittest" are at play here. The structures that can survive multiple turns are more likely to be present than those that are not. Over time, chance dictates they will eventually emerge.

Of course, these are not alive. Nor are they particularly complex or impressive.

What's also interesting, though, is what can be built by human hands.

If you decide to "rig the game" by creating the initial starting pattern (seed), then you can create structures designed to be self-sustaining. From there, you can leverage the rules of the game to create some incredible automation.

Examples include working calculators and even computers. The latter means that *Life* is "Turing Complete." In other words, you could theoretically build anything in *Life* that you could build with any given computer.

Yes, you could get *Doom* running in Life.

You can also build a simulation of Conway's *Life* within *Life*![77]

Now imagine a huge enough starting grid with the right number of starting cells and unlimited turns. Eventually, sheer probability would likely dictate that these structures would occur "naturally."

Just as we believe a monkey hitting keys at random on a typewriter for an infinite amount of time would eventually produce the complete works of Shakespeare.

Given that possibility, and the process of natural selection at play, is it possible we could *eventually* see the rise of an intelligent being?

Something entirely alien to us but capable of intelligent thought? Reproduction? Further evolution?

Of course, this is a thought experiment and likely wouldn't work (it requires a materialistic view of consciousness). Most starting seeds are ultimately self-limiting. And we currently lack powerful enough hardware to mimic the near-infinite scope needed for such a simulation.

I also believe an element of chance would need to be injected into the rules to better simulate our universal laws.

This is speculation on my part, but without an element of chance, you create no *new* information from The Game of Life. After all: the ending state could be extrapolated from the starting state.

---

77   Is the brain Turing complete? That's a complicated question.

The random "birth" of new cells would also allow for greater stability of seeds. Don't think this is new stuff; people have experimented with the rules of Life and many similar programs ad-nauseum.

Currently, we cannot build machines capable of producing truly random numbers. This, I believe, is truly limiting our ability to create any form of "life."

Similarly, it is the predictable "flow-chart thinking" that gives away most AI during a Turing test.[78]

But that's a thought experiment for another time.

The point I wanted to make here is if any of this theorizing is correct, the chances are that we *too* emerged from our environment in this way.

Our environment can be represented as a huge data set: a series of numbers and algorithms. We are one such algorithm. I believe we were forged *by* the environment around us.

As we continue to be.

---

78 This is what I think about when I'm on the toilet.

CONCLUSION AND CLOSING THOUGHTS

Okay, that was pretty out there.

So, let's return to reality for a moment.

Ultimately, the big takeaway is that the human body is incredibly adaptable. Our job is to provide the right stimulus to ensure that adaptation is positive.

This is a job we have largely been failing at. Miserably.

But by moving more throughout the day. By remembering the specific movements that we evolved for. By training in a more dynamic, unpredictable fashion. By constantly learning and changing… We can reclaim our original dynamism and adaptability.

I hope I've been able to outline a few practical ways of achieving this: through Vector Sets and incidental training, by training outdoors and with more unruly tools.

And we must remember that the goal is not to look like an inhuman, muscle-bound creature. Nor is it to simply be able to lift an extreme amount of weight in one constrained movement pattern.

Saying you want to work purely on your strength and not worry about mobility is like saying you want to look after your teeth and not your nails.

The human body is endlessly complex, but fortunately, we don't need to understand it to train it. We simply nourish it with regular movement and the right amount of challenge.

Good luck out there; thanks for reading...

And bye for now!

ABOUT THE AUTHOR

Adam Sinicki, a.k.a. The Bioneer, is a fitness/self-improvement YouTuber. He has a personal training diploma and BSc in Psychology. His YouTube channel has 474,000 subscribers and his Instagram has 25,500 followers. His previous book *Functional Training and Beyond* has a 4.7-star rating with over 681 reviews.

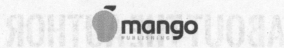

Mango Publishing, established in 2014, publishes an eclectic list of books by diverse authors—both new and established voices—on topics ranging from business, personal growth, women's empowerment, LGBTQ+ studies, health, and spirituality to history, popular culture, time management, decluttering, lifestyle, mental wellness, aging, and sustainable living. We were recently named 2019 *and* 2020's #1 fastest-growing independent publisher by *Publishers Weekly*. Our success is driven by our main goal, which is to publish high-quality books that will entertain readers as well as make a positive difference in their lives.

Our readers are our most important resource; we value your input, suggestions, and ideas. We'd love to hear from you—after all, we are publishing books for you!

Please stay in touch with us and follow us at:

Facebook: Mango Publishing
Twitter: @MangoPublishing
Instagram: @MangoPublishing
LinkedIn: Mango Publishing
Pinterest: Mango Publishing

Newsletter: mangopublishinggroup.com/newsletter

Join us on Mango's journey to reinvent publishing, one book at a time.